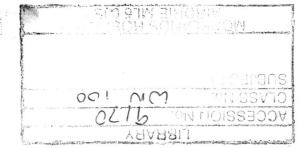

Radiology for Anaesthesia and

Radiology for Anaesthesia and Intensive Care

Richard Hopkins
Consultant Radiologist
Department of Radiology
Cheltenham General Hospital

Carol Peden
Consultant Anaesthetist
Royal Bath United Hospital

Sanjay Gandhi
Department of Clinical Radiology
Bristol Royal Infirmary

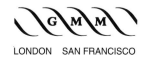

LONDON   SAN FRANCISCO

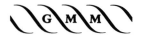

Greenwich Medical Media
4th Floor, 137 Euston Road,
London
NW1 2AA

© 2003

870 Market Street, Ste 720
San Francisco
CA 94109, USA

ISBN   184110 1192

First published 2003

www.greenwich-medical.co.uk

Distributed worldwide by Plymbridge Distributors Ltd and
in the USA by Jamco Distribution

Typeset by Charon Tec Pvt. Ltd, Chennai, India

Printed by The Alden Group Ltd, Oxford

Contents

Contents

Acknowledgements

Contributions to the book have been made by Dr I. Taylor, Dr C. Cook, Dr C. Styles, Dr D. Fox and Dr R. Lowe.

All images contributed by Dr R. Hopkins and Dr S. Gandhi unless otherwise stated.

Further images contributed by

Chapter 1
Mr L. Marchenco (Figs 1.1–1.4)
Dr M. Thornton (Fig. 1.48)
Dr M. O'Driscoll (Fig 1.53)
Dr M. Darby (Figs 1.55, 1.78, 1.83)
Dr J. Hawarth (Figs 1.80–1.82, 1.84–1.86)

Chapter 2
Dr A. Chalmers and Bath Royal United Hospital Film Museum
(Figs 2.11, 2.14, 2.15, 2.18, 2.19, 2.28)
Mr R. Law (Figs 2.24–2.27)
Dr N. Slack (Figs 2.33–2.35)
Dr M. Gibson (Fig. 2.36)

Chapter 4
Dr D. Graeb, Dr N. Müller (Figs 4.23, 4.24)
Vancouver General Hospital Department of Radiology

Chapter 6
Dr M. O'Driscoll (Fig. 6.14)

Contributors

Lai Peng Chan
Vancouver General Hospital
British Columbia
Canada

Richard Gee
Vancouver General Hospital
British Columbia
Canada

Cieran Keogh
Vancouver General Hospital
British Columbia
Canada

Nicola Matcham
Specialist Registrar in Radiology
Bristol Royal Infirmary
Bristol, UK

Peter Munk
Vancouver General Hospital
British Columbia
Canada

Savvas Nicolaou
Vancouver General Hospital
British Columbia
Canada

James K. Ralph
Specialist Registrar in Anaesthesia
University Department of Anaesthesia
The Queen Elizabeth Hospital
Birmingham, UK

Introduction

This book has been written for anaesthetists and intensive care doctors working in hospital practice. The material in the book covers all the common pathologies encountered in hospital anaesthetic practice and intensive care. Included are the core radiological requirements for the FRCA examination, but it is also ideally suited for doctors preparing for the Diploma in Intensive Care Medicine. It is not only intended as an examination revision aid, but also as a general radiological or revision text in anaesthetic radiology. In addition to the more commonly encountered areas such as chest and abdominal imaging, particular attention has been given to the topics of cervical spine imaging and blunt trauma. Sections covering trauma imaging of the chest, abdomen, pelvis, cervical-spine and head are included.

An excellent knowledge of anatomy is crucial when interpreting any radiological investigation. Particular attention has been paid to illustrating relevant radiological anatomy. For each body system (chest and cardiovascular, abdomen and pelvis, and head), the radiological anatomy of both conventional radiographs and CT is discussed in some detail. This appears at the beginning of the relevant chapters. For instance Chapter 1, *Imaging the chest*, includes detailed diagrams of the cardiac silhouette, the mediastinal outline and the anatomy which appears on a conventional chest radiograph. In addition, the anatomy visible on chest CT is explained and illustrated. Technology in radiology is advancing rapidly especially in the fields of cross-sectional imaging such as CT and MRI. Clinicians require a basic understanding of how various imaging modalities work in order to be able to interpret the images correctly. The basic principles of image formation in CT, MRI and ultrasound are explained. These imaging modalities are of particular relevance to anaesthetists as they frequently accompany sick patients to radiology departments for clinical imaging studies. Special attention is paid to the unique problems encountered in MRI scanners with particular regard to patient monitoring and support systems.

In radiology, a diagnosis is often made by recognising patterns of disease. Various imaging patterns such as air space shadowing, interstitial lung patterns, solitary or multiple pulmonary nodules, etc. often have a broad differential diagnosis. Final diagnosis is dependent upon clinical history, imaging features and further laboratory investigations. The clinical case scenarios in the book have been written to include clinical history, results of investigations and the radiology. For each case, a differential diagnosis is given where appropriate and anaesthetic management is discussed.

To derive the maximum benefit from each chapter, it is recommended that the introduction to the main chapters is read prior to attempting the accompanying clinical cases.

About the FRCA examination

James K. Ralph, Carol J. Peden

The Diploma of Fellow of the Royal College of Anaesthetists is a
two-part examination. These two parts are known as the Primary and Final
examinations. Each part comprises both written and viva examinations,
with the Primary also including an 'OSCE' (Objective Structured Clinical
Examination).

The Primary examination

The Primary examination is designed to assess trainees who have
completed 12 months of recognised training, although most will have
completed 18 months, before attempting the examination. The Primary
examination examines both the relevant basic sciences and clinical
practice of anaesthesia undertaken in the 12–18 months of training.
Candidates are expected to demonstrate a good understanding of the
fundamentals of clinical anaesthesia practice. With particular reference
to radiology, this includes the selection and interpretation of relevant
pre-operative investigations. Radiological images that may be encountered
will appear in the OSCE section of the examination. Interpretation will
take the form of short questions based on chest radiographs, neck and
thoracic inlet films, abdominal fluid levels/air/masses, skull films and other
imaging investigations (simple data only). The clinical viva in the Primary
examination does not include X-ray interpretation.

The Final examination

The Final examination is designed to assess trainees who have passed
the Primary examination and completed a minimum of 30 months of
recognised training. Final examination candidates are expected to have a
thorough knowledge of medicine and surgery, appropriate to the practice
of anaesthesia, intensive care and pain management. This includes
pre-operative assessment and selection and interpretation of appropriate
investigations. It also includes knowledge of diagnostic imaging and

the appropriate anaesthesia and sedation, preanaesthetic preparation and techniques appropriate for adults and children for CT scan, MRI and angiography and post-investigation care. An understanding of the principles of imaging techniques including CT, MRI and ultrasound is also required.

The Final examination is also divided into four parts: MCQ, SAQ and two vivas. There are two structured vivas: Viva 1 (50 minutes) – Clinical Anaesthesia – is where radiological images will occur. This viva consists of a long case and three short cases. During the first 10 minutes, you will have the opportunity to view on your own clinical information related to the long case, including radiological images (usually a chest X-ray). There are easy marks to be had if you have practised X-ray interpretation. An ordered, sensible approach to the chest X-ray will also give the examiners the impression that you are safe and experienced – practise and impress them! During the final 20 minutes you will be asked questions on three further clinical topics.

Preparation

Preparation for the examination should start by obtaining and reading the current syllabus and the examination regulations, which can be obtained from the College. A period of intensive study is a prerequisite to success but also realistic viva practice from consultant colleagues and recent successful examination candidates. It is important to develop a system for reviewing and presenting X-rays and again, practise with colleagues, and preferably a radiologist, will refine your technique.

Competency-based training and assessment

Becoming a safe and competent anaesthetist is not only about passing the appropriate examinations; workplace assessments must be successfully completed by an SHO to achieve the SHO training certificate in order to apply for an SpR post. An SpR must pass the appropriate competency tests in order to receive accreditation. An SHO must be able to interpret simple radiological images showing clear abnormalities including chest radiographs, CT and MRI scans of head, neck and thoracic inlet films, and films showing abdominal fluid levels/air. At SpR level, the anaesthetist should understand the implications of different radiological procedures in their anaesthetic care of the patient and be able to establish safe anaesthesia or sedation within the confines and limitations of the X-ray department.

Recommended reading

Primary and Final Examinations for the FRCA – Syllabus. Royal College of Anaesthetists, March 2000 (ISBN 1 900936 755).

Primary and Final Examinations for the FRCA – Regulations. Royal College of Anaesthetists, January 2002 (ISBN 1 900936 16X).

The CCST in Anaesthesia. Manuals for trainees and trainers, Parts I–III. Royal College of Anaesthetists, 2000–2002.

RCA website: http://www.rcoa.ac.uk

The Royal College of Anaesthesists Guide to the Primary FRCA Examination. The Primary. Ed. Paul Cartwright. Royal College of Anaesthetists, 2001.

The Clinical Anaesthesia Viva Book. Eds. Mills S.J., Maguire S.L., Barker J.M. Greenwich Medical Media, London, 2002.

The pre-operative assessment

James K. Ralph

Looking at X-ray films as part of the pre-operative assessment

Pre-operative assessment consists of the consideration of information from multiple sources that may include the patient's medical record, interview, physical examination and findings from medical tests and evaluations. Pre-operative tests may be indicated for various purposes including:

- discovery or identification of a disease or disorder which may affect peri-operative anaesthetic care;
- verification or assessment of an already known disease, disorder or therapy;
- formulation of specific plans and alternatives for peri-operative care.

Any test required for a patient should be ordered with the reasonable expectation that it will result in benefit, such as a change in the timing or selection of a technique or appropriate pre-operative optimisation, that exceeds any potential adverse effects.

A number of guidelines and publications by various working parties and taskforces exist with advice on which investigations are appropriate, when they are appropriate and in which individuals.

Association of Anaesthetists of Great Britain and Ireland [1]

Blanket routine pre-operative investigations are inefficient, expensive and unnecessary. Medical and anaesthetic problems are identified more efficiently by the taking of a history and by the physical examination of patients. It should be remembered that pre-operative investigations can themselves be the cause of morbidity.

Departments should have policies on which investigations should be performed. These should reflect the patients' age, co-morbidity and the complexity of surgery. Chest X-rays should be arranged in accordance with the recommendations from the Royal College of Radiologists in conjunction with local hospital policy.

Royal College of Radiologists [2]

The pre-operative chest X-ray is not routinely indicated. Exceptions are before cardio-pulmonary surgery, likely admission to ITU, suspected malignancy or TB. Anaesthetists may also request chest X-rays for dyspnoeic patients, those with known cardiac disease and the very elderly. Many patients with cardio-respiratory disease have a recent chest X-ray available; a repeat chest X-ray is not then usually required.

Task Force on Preanaesthetic Evaluation of the American Society of Anaesthesiologists [3]

The Task Force 'agreed that pre-operative tests including chest X-ray should not be ordered routinely. The Task Force agreed that pre-operative tests might be performed on a selective basis for the purpose of guiding or optimising management …'.

'The Task Force agreed that the clinical characteristics to consider when deciding whether to order a pre-operative chest X-ray include smoking, recent upper respiratory tract infection (URTI), chronic obstructive pulmonary disease (COPD) and cardiac disease. The Task Force agreed chest X-ray abnormalities may be higher in such patients but does not believe that extremes of age, smoking, stable COPD, stable cardiac disease or recent resolved URTI should be considered unequivocal indications for chest X-ray.'

In their review of the literature, they noted that routine chest X-rays were reported as abnormal in 2.5–60.1% of cases (20 studies) and led to changes in management in 0–51% of cases found to be abnormal (9 studies). Indicated chest X-rays were reported as abnormal in 7.7–65.4% of cases (18 studies) and led to a change in management in 0.5–74% of cases (9 studies). In other words, there is a wide range of reported abnormality in both routine and indicated chest X-ray many of which do not result in a change in patient management.

In summary, the routine pre-operative chest X-ray is not routinely indicated. It should be preceded by a thorough history and physical examination and ordered if these elicit an indication consistent with departmental policies in conjunction with recommendations from the Royal College of Radiologists. This should result in requests for chest X-rays that have a higher probability of showing an abnormality, which will then be acted on with a change in patient management whilst minimizing risk to the patient.

References

1. Preoperative Assessment. The Role of the Anaesthetist. Association of Anaesthetists of Great Britain and Ireland, 2001.
2. Making the Best Use of a Department of Clinical Radiology: Guidelines for Doctors, 4th edition. Royal College of Radiologists, 1998 (ISBN 1872599370).
3. Practice Advisory for Preanaesthetic Evaluation. A Report by the American Society of Anaesthesiologists Task Force on Preanaesthetic Evaluation, 2001.

Imaging the chest

How to read a chest X-ray

Reading a chest X-ray requires a methodical approach that can be applied to all films so that abnormalities are not overlooked. Clinicians and radiologists develop an individual approach but there are certain core areas that should be looked at on all films. These may be inspected in any order – this is largely down to personal preference. Listed below is the outline of a method which can be applied to read chest X-rays.

Initial quick review of film
To identify any obvious abnormality.

Systematic analysis

Label
Verify the patient's identity. In examination situations look at the name, if present, as this can give a clue to sex and ethnic background.
The date and hospital where the film was taken give further clues. If a film has been taken at a centre for oncology or chest medicine, for instance, this may help with interpretation.

Projection and patient position
Postero-anterior (PA) is the preferred projection as this does not produce as much radiographic magnification of the heart and mediastinum as an antero-posterior (AP) projection. A PA film is taken with the film cassette in front of the patient and the beam delivered from behind with the patient in an upright position. Portable films and those taken on intensive care are all AP projection. Patient position causes important although sometimes subtle variations in appearance. The supine position causes distension of the upper lobe blood vessels which may be confused with elevated left atrial pressure. Imaging of a pleural effusion in a supine position appears as faint increased density over a hemithorax – this is due to fluid collecting in the dependent part of the chest, i.e. as a thin layer posteriorly.

All films taken in the AP projection are usually labelled as such but to avoid difficulties when describing films in examinations the use of the term frontal projection is often helpful.

A lateral radiograph is used to localise lesions in the AP dimension; locate lesions behind the left side of the heart or in the posterior recesses of the lungs. A left lateral (with the left side of the chest against the film and the beam projected from the right) is the standard projection. The heart is magnified less with a left lateral as it is closer to the film. To visualise lesions in the left thorax obtain a left lateral film and for right-sided lesions a right lateral.

Lordotic views are taken to examine the lung apices if potential lesions are partially obscured by overlying ribs or the clavicles. This view was formerly taken in an AP position with the patient leaning backwards by

30 degrees. Now they are obtained in a PA position with the beam angled downward by 45 degrees – a less awkward position for patients.

Expiratory films are used to assess air trapping in bronchial obstruction such as a foreign body. A pneumothorax always appears larger on an expiratory film and occasionally a small pneumothorax may only be visible on expiration.

Side marker
Dextrocardia is easily missed if the side marker is not identified.

Quality of film
- *Penetration* – the vertebral bodies should just be visible through the cardiac silhouette.

- *Rotation* – the medial aspect of the clavicles should be symmetrically positioned on either side of the spine.

- *Inspiration* – the diaphragm should lie at the level of the sixth or seventh rib anteriorly.

Large airways, lungs and pleura
The 'lung shadows' are composed of the pulmonary arteries and veins. Apart from the pulmonary vessels, the lungs should appear black because they contain air. Examine the lungs for density variation. Compare the interspaces on the right with those on the left. Compare the right side with the left just as you would, if auscultating the chest. Look all the way out to the periphery of the lungs. Look at the overall lung vascularity and compare one side with the other. It is important to look at the main airways – the trachea and the main bronchi. Check the position of the trachea, that it is central and not deviated.

Look at the pleural surfaces and the fissures, if visible. Check for masses, calcifications fluid or pneumothorax.

Heart and mediastinum
Examine the cardiac outline identifying all the heart borders and the outline of the great vessels (see Figs 1.1 and 1.2). Check that there are not any abnormal densities projected through the cardiac silhouette. Look at the aortic and pulmonary artery outlines. The heart and mediastinal outline are made up of a series of 'bumps' (see Fig. 1.3). On the right side, there are right braciocephalic vessels, the ascending aorta and superior vena cava, the right atrium, and the inferior vena cava. On the left side, there are four 'moguls' in addition to the left brachiocephalic vessels: these are the aortic arch, the pulmonary trunk, the left atrial appendage and the left ventricle. The size and shape of each of these structures need to be looked at for signs of enlargement or reduction in size. The right heart border is created by the right atrium alone (the right ventricle is an anterior structure, therefore does not contribute to any heart borders) – this is a question examiners love to ask (see Fig. 1.4).

1

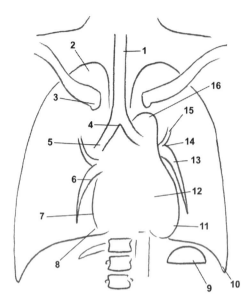

Fig. 1.1 Diagram of normal frontal chest X-ray: 1. trachea, 2. right lung apex, 3. clavicle, 4. carina, 5. right main bronchus, 6. right lower lobe pulmonary artery, 7. right artium, 8. right cardiophrenic angle, 9. gastric air bubble, 10. costophrenic angle, 11. left ventricle, 12. descending thoracic aorta, 13. left lower lobe pulmonary artery, 14. left hilum, 15. left upper lobe pulmonary vein, 16. aortic arch.

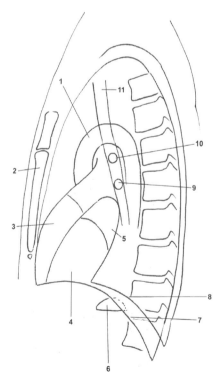

Fig. 1.2 Diagram of normal lateral chest X-ray: 1. ascending thoracic aorta, 2. sternum, 3. right ventricle, 4. left ventricle, 5. left atrium, 6. gastric air bubble, 7. right hemidiaphragm, 8. left hemidiaphragm, 9. right upper lobe bronchus, 10. left upper lobe bronchus, 11. trachea.

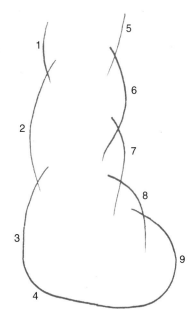

Fig. 1.3 The 'bumps' which make up the cardiac silhouette: 1. right brachiocephalic vein, 2. ascending aorta and superimposed SVC, 3. right atrium, 4. inferior vena cava, 5. left brachiocephalic vessels, 6. aortic arch, 7. pulmonary trunk, 8. left atrial appendage, 9. left ventricle.

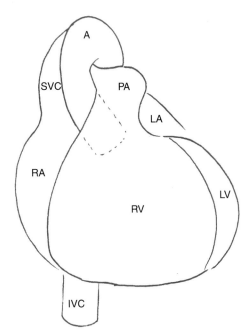

Fig. 1.4 Cardiac chambers and great vessels: LA, left atrial appendage; RA, right atrium; LV, left ventricle; RV, right ventricle; IVC, inferior vena cava; SVC, superior vena cava; PA, pulmonary artery; A, ascending aorta.

Heart size can be estimated using the cardiothoracic ratio. The cardiac measurement is taken as the greatest transverse heart diameter and is compared to the greatest internal width of the thorax. A ratio of greater than 0.5 is often used in clinical practice to indicate cardiomegaly.

Look at the position of the hila and their density – compare the left with the right side. Tumours and enlarged lymph nodes can occur here making the hila appear bulky.

Diaphragm

Check the shape, position and clarity/sharpness of both hemidiaphragms. Both costophrenic angles should be clear and sharp. The cardiophrenic angles should be fairly clear – cardiophrenic fat pads can cause added density. The right hemidiaphragm is usually slightly higher than the left – up to 1.5 cm. On the lateral film, the right hemidiaphragm is seen in its entirety but the anterior aspect of the left hemidiaphragm merges with the heart, so is not seen (see Fig. 1.6).

Bones

This is an area which is frequently overlooked.

- *Ribs*: The ribs are a common site for fracture or metastatic deposits but the remainder of the skeleton must also be carefully examined. Identify the first rib and carefully trace its contour from the spine to its junction with the manubrium. Each rib must be carefully and individually traced in this manner, initially for one hemithorax and then the contralateral side. A useful trick is to turn the film on its side, rib fractures may then appear more obvious.

- *Thoracic spine*: Look at the thoracic spine alignment – is it straight or is there a scoliosis? Take particular care to exclude pathology from the thoracic spine in trauma patients when even moderate malalignment can be overlooked when projected through the heart or mediastinal shadows.

- *Clavicles scapulae and humeri*: Fractures and dislocation of the humerus are often obvious when looked for. Look for fractures, metastatic deposits, abnormal calcifications or evidence of arthritis around the shoulders.

Soft tissues

A visual examination should be routinely performed on the chest wall, the neck and both the breast shadows. Look for surgical emphysema and abnormal calcification. With reference to the breast shadows be sure to check whether there are two breast shadows and whether there is symmetry of size, shape and position. The lung field missing a breast will appear a little darker than the other side.

Review areas

These review areas are sites where pathology is commonly missed and warrant a second look before any chest X-ray is reported as normal:

- Breasts (symmetry/mastectomy).

- Below the diaphragm, do not forget that the lungs extend below the diaphragms, also look at the upper abdomen for surgical clips/calcification/pneumoperitoneum.

- Behind the heart (hiatus hernia/lung nodules/left lower lobe collapse).
- Thoracic spine and paraspinal lines (trauma).
- Clavicle (nodule behind medial end and eroded lateral end).
- Shoulder (dislocation).
- Apices (pancoast tumour).
- Hila (assess position, size and density).
- Lung parenchyma.
- Bones, especially ribs (look for metastases or fractures).

The 'normal' chest X-ray in examination vivas

Hopefully the situation, i.e. when you are unable to spot an abnormality on the film will not arise (in a viva). In a viva-type situation, the examiner has chosen a normal looking film because the findings are subtle and he/she is assessing whether you have a systematic approach. There are certain diagnoses which are easily made if you remember to look. A list of these is given below. It can be worth specifically looking for these, if no abnormality is immediately apparent as it creates a bad impression if you miss something elementary like a left lower lobe collapse. If the film looks normal, check the review areas again. This not only helps to pass examination vivas but is also a good clinical practice and will improve your day-to-day assessment of chest X-rays.

In particular look for

- dextrocardia,
- mastectomy,
- left lower lobe collapse,
- pneumothorax,
- middle lobe collapse.

Films that frequently appear in the anaesthetic clinical viva include: pneumothoraces, lobar collapse/consolidation, ARDS, enlarged heart (mitral stenosis, hypertension, cardiomyopathy), pulmonary hypertension and oedema, flail chest/contusion injury, COPD, pleural effusion, severe kyphoscoliosis and enlarged thyroid with tracheal deviation!

Having looked at the chest X-ray, it remains to classify the signs into a radiographic pattern. Particular radiographic patterns have a list of diagnostic possibilities. Radiographic patterns include: consolidation, interstitial shadowing, nodules, pleural disease, mediastinal masses, etc. The case examples systematically discuss many of the more commonly encountered radiographic patterns encountered in anaesthetic practice or on intensive care units. Short lists of differential diagnoses are given in the following case examples.

Case illustrations: plain films and CT

Question 1

■ Name the structures labelled on these chest X-rays (Figs 1.5 and 1.6).

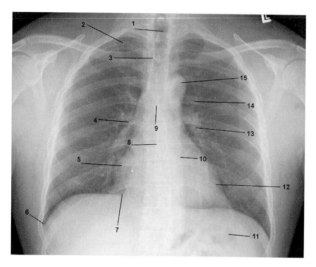

Fig. 1.5 Quiz case.

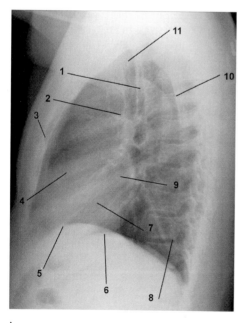

Fig. 1.6 Quiz case.

Answer (Fig. 1.5)

1. Trachea
2. Lung apex
3. Right para-tracheal stripe
4. Right hilum
5. Right atrium (not ventricle!)
6. Right costophrenic angle
7. Right cardiophrenic angle
8. Azygo-oesophageal stripe
9. Carina
10. Descending thoracic aorta
11. Gastric air bubble
12. Left ventricle
13. Left lower lobe pulmonary artery
14. Left upper lobe pulmonary vein
15. Aortic arch

Answer (Fig. 1.6)

1. Trachea
2. Aortopulmonary window
3. Sternum
4. Right ventricle
5. Right hemidiaphragm
6. Left hemidiaphragm
7. Left ventricle
8. Posterior recess of lung
9. Left atrium
10. Scapula
11. Lung apex

Question 2

■ Name the structures on these chest CT scans (Figs. 1.7–1.10).

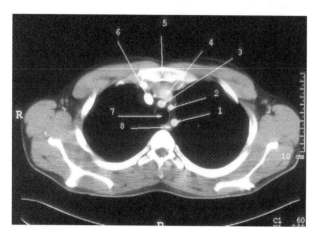

Fig. 1.7 Quiz case.

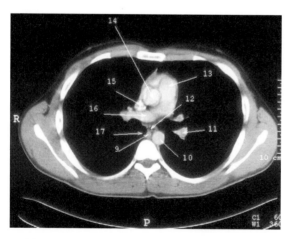

Fig. 1.8 Quiz case.

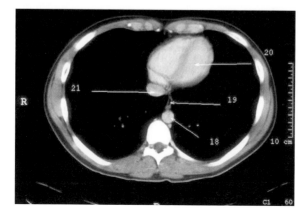

Fig. 1.9 Quiz case.

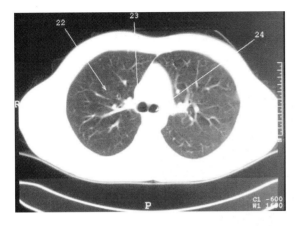

Fig. 1.10 Quiz case.

Answer (Figs 1.7–1.10)

1. Left subclavian artery
2. Left common carotid artery
3. Brachiocephalic artery
4. Left brachiocephalic vein
5. Sternum
6. Superior vena cava (SVC)
7. Trachea
8. Oesophagus
9. Azygous vein
10. Descending aorta
11. Left lower lobe pulmonary artery
12. Oesophagus
13. Main pulmonary artery
14. Aortic root
15. SVC
16. Right pulmonary artery
17. Azygo-oesophageal recess
18. Descending aorta
19. Oesophagus
20. Left ventricle
21. Inferior vena cava (IVC)
22. Right lung (upper lobe)
23. Mediastinum
24. Left main bronchus

Question 3

34-year-old male.
Pleuritic chest pain. Short of breath.

■ What is the diagnosis (Fig. 1.11)?

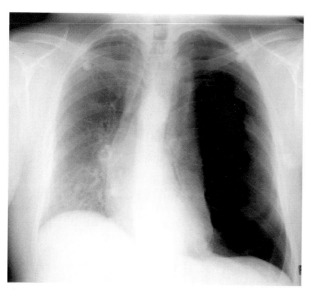

Fig. 1.11 Quiz case.

Answer

Tension pneumothorax

There is a large left-sided tension pneumothorax with mediastinal shift to the right side and depression of the left hemidiaphragm. A chest drain needs to be inserted urgently.

In supine patients, beware of skin folds which can simulate pneumothorax – these can sometimes be followed beyond the chest wall. In normal lung, the vasculature cannot be seen in the peripheral 1–2 cm and the absence of pulmonary vasculature is only a secondary sign of pneumothorax. In a supine patient, air collects anteriorly often adjacent to the cardiac silhouette causing it to appear sharper than usual (see Fig. 1.12). Supine pneumothorax is commonly seen in the intensive care setting because patients are X-rayed supine and if there is co-existent respiratory distress, then the lungs are 'stiffer' and fail to collapse.

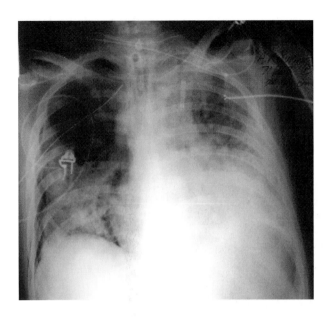

Fig. 1.12 Supine pneumothorax. The patient is on intensive care, has a tracheostomy and various lines. The right heart border is 'too' clearly seen because it is outlined by air.

Question 4

24-year-old patient living in home for educational special needs. Breathless and distressed.

- What do the chest X-rays (Fig. 1.13, inspiration; Fig. 1.14, expiration) show?
- What is the management?

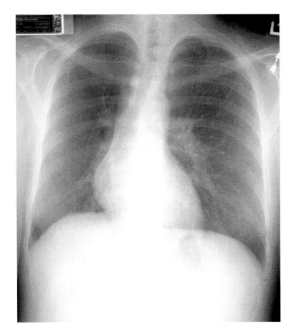

Fig. 1.13 Quiz case.

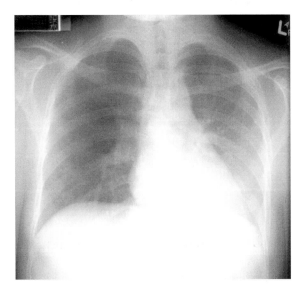

Fig. 1.14 Quiz case.

Answer

Aspiration of foreign body

The films are taken in inspiration and expiration giving the clue that the suspected diagnosis is an inhaled foreign body. The inspiratory film shows loss of volume of the right hemithorax with shift of the mediastinum to the right. On the expiratory film, there is air trapping on the affected side as the foreign body has prevented complete expiration from the right lung. If the film is examined carefully, there is an opacity in the right main bronchus which is an inhaled foreign body.

Management involves bronchoscopy, either rigid or flexibly and extraction of the foreign body. Forceps, baskets and fogarty balloons can be used to try and grasp the foreign body.

Endobronchial foreign body

Aspiration of a foreign body can be a life-threatening event. If the object is large enough to occlude the airway, death can rapidly occur from asphyxia. Most foreign bodies are radiolucent, so air trapping or atelectasis may be the only sign. Atelectasis may not develop for 24 hours. CT is an alternative imaging method if chest X-ray is non-diagnostic or fluoroscopy to observe diaphragmatic and mediastinal shifts due to air trapping.

The commonest age group is 16 and below, particularly age 1–3. Commonly aspirated objects include nuts, seeds, bone fragments, small toys, food or teeth (Figs 1.15 and 1.16). Until the age of 15, the angles made by the mainstem bronchi with the trachea are equal, so aspiration is equally likely into either bronchus. With age, the right mainstem bronchus makes a straighter course from the larynx and trachea so after the age of 15 objects are more often found on the right side.

Symptoms include cough, wheeze, stridor, dyspnoea and cyanosis. Organic foreign bodies can swell or induce an inflammatory response with granulation tissue. Swelling and bleeding can make removal difficult.

Complications include:

- mediastinitis,
- air trapping/local emphysema,
- atelectasis/lobar collapse,
- post-obstruction pneumonia,
- abscess,
- bronchiectasis,
- stricture formation.

Complications are reduced with prompt extraction (less than 24 hours). Anaesthetic management of the small child who has inhaled a foreign body is a common examination question.

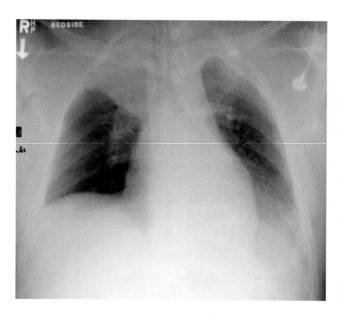

Fig. 1.15 Aspirated and swallowed teeth following facial trauma. Right upper lobe collapse and partial collapse of left lower lobe. Opacities in the stomach.

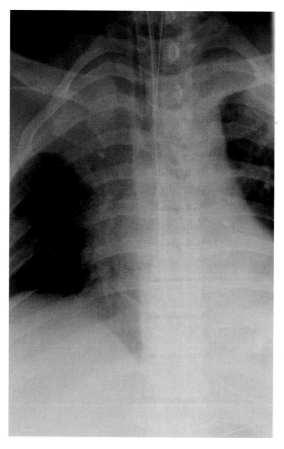

Fig. 1.16 The penetrated film demonstrates tooth fragments in the right upper lobe bronchus and also the left lower lobe bronchus.

Question 5

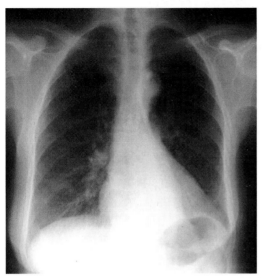

72-year-old smoker.
Haemoptysis and cough.

■ What does the chest X-ray (Fig. 1.17) show?

Fig. 1.17 Quiz case.

Answer

Left lower lobe collapse

Lobar or segmental collapse occurs in large airway obstruction and subsequent absorbtion of air from the affected lung. Causes are listed below. Bronchogenic malignancy is one of the commonest causes and the case study illustrates the subtle signs on plain X-ray. Subsequent CT imaging of this patient demonstrated a malignant neoplasm originating in the left lower lobe bronchus.

Table 1.1 **Causes of lobar collapse**

■ Luminal mass
  ● Neoplasm (carcinoma, carcinoid)
  ● Foreign body (peanut) (see Figs 1.15 and 1.16)
  ● Mucus plug/inflammatory exudate
  ● Endoluminal metastasis
  ● Misplaced endotracheal tube (ITU ventilated patients)

■ Bronchial wall
  ● Inflammation (TB, sarcoid)

■ Extrinsic compression
  ● Lymph nodes
  ● aneurysm

1

In children, bronchial malignancy is rare and the causes of lobar collapse differ from those in adults. Inflammatory exudate in pneumonia or mucus plugging (in patients with cystic fibrosis and asthma) are much more common causes (Table 1.1).

The five lobes collapse in different directions to produce different patterns although there are some common features (see below). If the vessels within the collapsed lobe remain perfused, then a wedge-shaped opacity is more clearly identified. In lower lobe collapse (both right and left lower lobe), the lung collapses posteriorly and medially. This is well illustrated by the CT scan (see Fig. 1.18). In left lower lobe collapse, the silhouette of the medial aspect of the hemidiaphragm and the descending

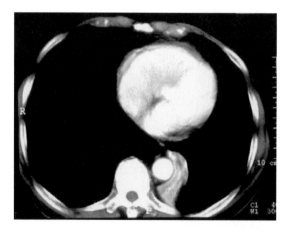

Fig. 1.18 CT left lower lobe collapse. Note how the left lower lobe collapses tight against the descending aorta.

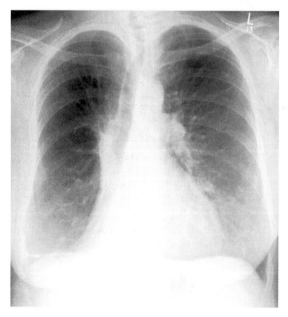

Fig. 1.19 Right lower lobe collapse. Loss of volume in the right lung, the right hemithorax is hypertranslucent.

aorta is lost because it is no longer outlined by adjacent aerated lung. A triangular opacity is seen projected through the cardiac outline. In right lower lobe collapse (Fig. 1.19), the hemidiaphragm silhouette remains clearly seen as the middle lobe is in contact with it. On a lateral projection the collapsed lower lobe may be identified as a triangle of increased density in the posterior costophrenic recess.

X-ray signs of lobar collapse
- Volume loss (hilar shift, mediastinal shift, hemidiaphragm elevation, rib crowding).
- Compensatory hyperinflation (translucency) of other lobes.
- Movement of fissures.
- Wedge-shaped opacity caused by collapsed lobe-specific pattern for each lobe.

Right upper lobe collapse
The right upper lobe collapses against the mediastinum and thoracic apex with a broad-based opacity radiating from the hilum. If there is an outward bulge at the right hilum, this is good evidence that a hilar mass is responsible for the collapse (see Fig. 1.20). The lower lobe pulmonary artery is pulled upwards and outwards.

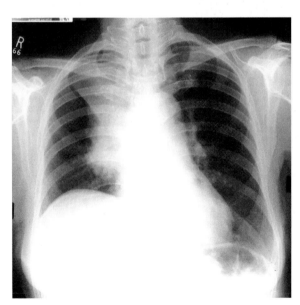

Fig. 1.20 Right upper lobe collapse. There is a mass at the right hilum which merges with the triangular opacity from the collapsed right upper lobe – 'Golden sign'. This 'S'-shaped appearance is typical of a neoplastic hilar mass responsible for the upper lobe collapse.

1

Left upper lobe collapse

This does not mirror right upper lobe collapse due to the absence of a middle lobe. The left upper lobe collapses forward against the anterior chest wall. The lower lobe expands behind it. The chest X-ray appearance is of a hazy density in the mid- and upper zones which fades away laterally and inferiorly (see Fig. 1.21). The collapsed lobe is adjacent to the left cardiac and mediastinal border, so this silhouette is completely lost. The aortic knuckle is lost (see Fig. 1.22) unless the lobar collapse is accompanied by overexpansion of the lower lobe with its superior segment occupying the apex.

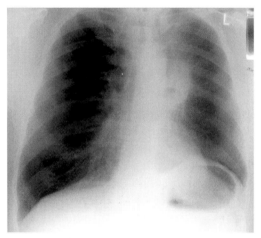

Fig. 1.21 Left upper lobe collapse.

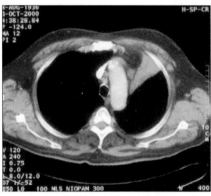
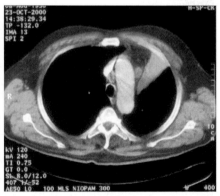

Fig. 1.22 Left upper lobe collapse CT. Note how the lobe collapses anteriorly against the chest wall.

Middle lobe collapse

This is easily missed on the frontal film and is often more obvious on a lateral projection. On the frontal projection, there is a vague increase in density seen in the right lower zone and the normally sharp right heart border is blurred. On a lateral projection the collapsed middle lobe forms a triangular opacity with its apex at the hilum and base projecting towards the sternum. (see Figs 1.23 and 1.24).

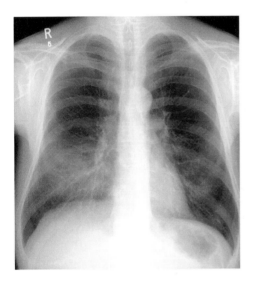

Fig. 1.23 Middle lobe collapse. Note the loss of outline of the right heart border.

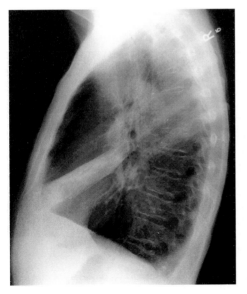

Fig. 1.24 Lateral projection middle lobe collapse. The triangular opacity is the collapsed middle lobe.

1

Question 6

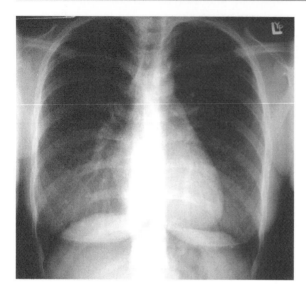

33-year-old man. Chest X-ray (Fig. 1.25) taken for purposes of obtaining a travel visa.

■ What are the findings?

Fig. 1.25 Quiz case.

Answer

Pectus excavatum

This chest wall deformity can simulate disease. The rib pairs are *heart shaped* and downward pointing in their lateral and anterior aspect. The heart is shifted to the left and superimposed soft tissue shadows at the right heart border create the impression of middle lobe disease. A lateral film will demonstrate the sternal depression and also confirm normality of the middle lobe. The CT (Fig. 1.26) demonstrates the thoracic cage deformity.

Other normal variants include cervical ribs, which are usually asymptomatic, but in a minority of cases individuals can be symptomatic with Raynauld's phenomenon. Distinction is made from normal transverse processes by the direction of slope. Cervical ribs slope downwards.

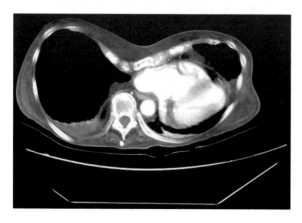

Fig. 1.26 CT pectus excavatum. Note the sternal depression and the movement of the heart to the left side.

Question 7

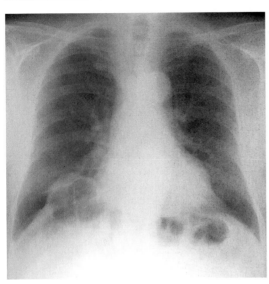

58-year-old man.
Abdominal pain.
Patient has a drug history
of corticosteroids use for
polymyalgia rheumatica.

- What does the X-ray
  (Fig. 1.27) show?

- Does the patient need
  laparotomy?

1

Fig. 1.27 Quiz case.

Answer

Diaphragmatic eventration and colonic interposition

This history is designed to mislead as no pathology is demonstrated here.
Interposition of colon between the liver and the diaphragm
(chilaiditis syndrome) can simulate pneumoperitoneum. Haustration of
the bowel can usually be identified but if there is doubt, then a left
lateral decubitus film should be performed.

In diaphragmatic eventration the normal muscular part of a
hemidiaphragm is deficient and replaced by connective tissue. There is
normally a dome-like bulging of the anterior aspect of the diaphragm.
It is common in the elderly when the bulging may be focal. A lateral
projection will show the posterior costophrenic recess to be in the normal
position and if screened under fluoroscopy some diaphragmatic movement
can be identified.

Question 8

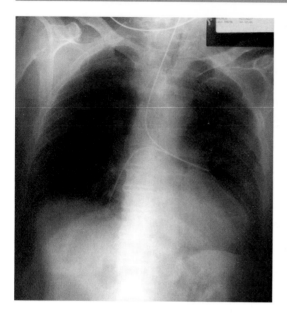

46-year-old patient on intensive care unit.

■ What does the chest X-ray (Fig. 1.28) show?

Fig. 1.28 Quiz case.

Answer

The tip of the nasogastric tube is in the right main bronchus and the more proximal part of the tube is coiled in the left main bronchus.

Checking the position of all tubes and lines is crucial for films taken on intensive care units. This should be done meticulously for each line by tracing it with the eye throughout its course.

Question 9

Chest X-ray (Fig. 1.29) taken prior to varicose vein surgery.

■ What is the diagnosis?

■ Are there any precautions necessary prior to anaesthesia?

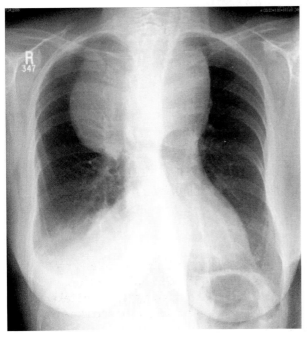

Fig. 1.29 Quiz case.

Answer

Retrosternal thyroid

This is the commonest cause of a superior mediastinal mass. It can displace and narrow the trachea and it frequently calcifies.

The patient should be euthyroid before elective surgery. Careful questioning, examination and thyroid function tests should be performed. If the mediastinal mass is compressing the trachea, then the patient may be symptomatic. If the tracheal diameter is reduced by more than 50%, then the patient will develop stridor, which may be positional or occur only on exercise. CT or MRI should be used to gain more information about the degree of tracheal compression. If significant, removal of the thyroid should take priority over elective varicose vein surgery. If there is no, or minimal, compression, then surgery may proceed. Regional block is an anaesthetic option.

Mediastinal masses

Mediastinal masses are classified according to their location in the mediastinum: anterior, middle and posterior mediastinum. It is possible to localise these with reasonable accuracy on plain films by assessing which silhouette has been lost. If, for example, part of the silhouette of the ascending thoracic aorta or heart border is blurred, then the mass must be anterior. If the lung hilum is seen projected through the mass and the hilum is of normal appearance, then the abnormality cannot be in the middle mediastinum. Posterior mediastinal masses are identified by the loss of the thoracic spine contour or the descending thoracic aorta outline. Other clues of a posteriorly sited mass are abnormalities of the adjacent ribs or bony involvement of the spine (see Fig. 1.30).

Lateral plain films will confirm the position in the mediastinum. Cross-sectional imaging (CT or MRI) are routinely used to give further anatomical detail of mediastinal masses (Table 1.2).

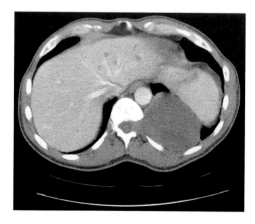

Fig. 1.30 Posterior mediastinal mass, a neurogenic tumour. It could be difficult to locate this mass in the posterior mediastinal on frontal chest X-ray – the clue to look for is the expansion of the neural foramina.

Table 1.2 **Mediastinal masses**

Anterior mediastinal masses – anatomical space anterior to trachea and major bronchi
- Thyroid
- Lymph nodes
- Thymic tumour (see Figs 1.31 and 1.32)
- Teratoma
- Ascending aortic aneurysm

Middle mediastinum – space between anterior and posterior mediastinum
- Lymph nodes (Fig. 1. 33)
- Aortic arch aneurysm
- Bronchogenic cyst

Posterior mediastinal mass – anatomical space posterior to anterior aspect of thoracic spine
- Hiatus hernia
- Lymph nodes
- Descending aortic aneurysm
- Neurogenic mass (Fig. 1.30)

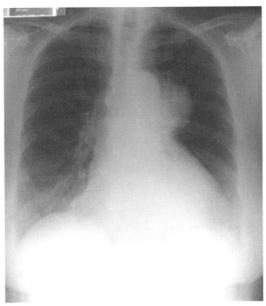

Fig. 1.31 Anterior mediastinal mass-thymoma. The mass blends into the aortic arch.

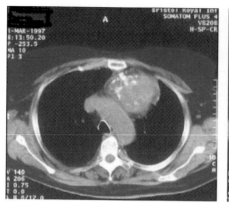
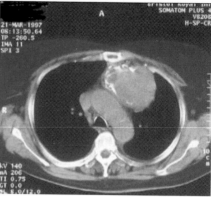

Fig. 1.32 CT thymoma. Cross-sectional imaging demonstrates the position of the mass in the anterior mediastinum.

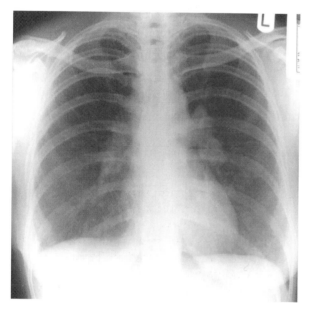

Fig. 1.33 Mass in the middle mediastinum. Bilateral hilar lymphadenopathy due to sarcoidosis.

Question 10

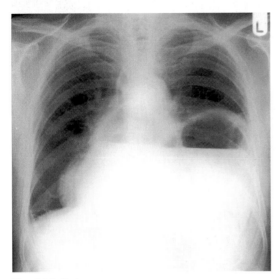

64-year-old patient
(Fig. 1.34).

■ What is the condition?

■ What anaesthetic
precautions are
necessary?

Fig. 1.34 Quiz case.

Answer

Hiatal hernia

A hiatal hernia is herniation of the stomach through the oesophageal
diaphragmatic hiatus into the thorax. The majority of hiatal hernias are
sliding, i.e. the gastro-oesophageal junction as well as part of the stomach
move up into the chest. The gastro-oesophageal junction remains correctly
located in a rolling hiatal hernia and part of the stomach herniates past it
up into the chest. Hiatal hernias are described as incarcerated when they
are irreducible. Hiatal hernias can be diagnosed on plain chest radiographs
where a gas shadow is seen projected through the cardiac silhouette.
If doubt exists, then a lateral projection can be performed (Fig. 1.35).
Hiatal hernias are a frequent finding on barium examinations of the upper
gastrointestinal tract.

1

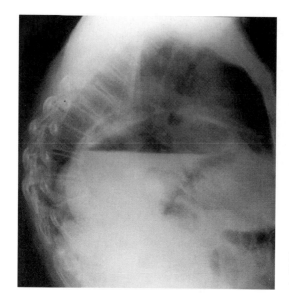

Fig. 1.35 Lateral projection of hiatus hernia. Note the air fluid levels in the stomach.

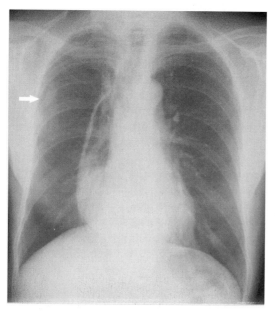

Fig. 1.36 Gastric pull-up. There has been an oesophagectomy and gastric pull-up procedure. The air fluid level is within the stomach. Note the right-sided rib changes from thoracotomy.

The appearance following oesophagectomy can also produce a large mediastinal gas shadow (sometimes with a fluid level) (see Fig. 1.36). Aspiration is a potential risk of general anaesthesia or sedation. Regional anaesthesia should be considered if appropriate for the surgery. The patient should be given an H_2 antagonist or proton pump inhibitor as pre-medication. If general anaesthesia is undertaken, a rapid sequence induction with cricoid pressure should be performed and the trachea intubated with a cuffed tube.

Question 11

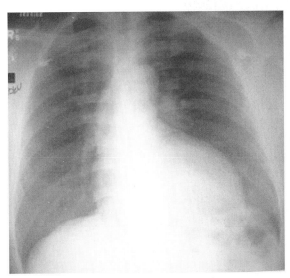

■ Report the chest X-ray (Fig. 1.37).

Fig. 1.37 Quiz case.

Answer

Aortic stenosis

There is cardiomegaly with a prominent ascending thoracic aorta and calcification in the region of the aortic valve. There is upper lobe blood diversion consistent with mild left ventricular failure.

Causes of aortic stenosis include congentital stenosis, a bicuspid aortic valve, rheumatic heart disease and senile calcific valve degeneration. The gradient across the heart valve produces left ventricular hypertrophy with increased muscle mass which can cause relative myocardial ischaemia and the risk of cardiac arrhythmias. If untreated, left ventricular decompensation leads to left ventricular dilatation and pulmonary venous congestion.

The X-ray findings include, post-stenotic dilatation of the aorta, calcification of the aortic valve and a left ventricular configuration seen at the left heart border with concavity along the mid-lateral border and increased convexity along the lower left heart border (Table 1.3).

Table 1.3 Causes of cardiomegaly

- Ischaemic heart disease
- Valvular heart disease
- Congenital heart disease
- Dilated cardiomyopathy
  - Viral
  - Alcohol (Fig. 1.38)
  - Metabolic
- Pericardial effusions

In left ventricular hypertrophy from hypertension or aortic stenosis, the cardiac silhouette does not dilate until late in the natural history.

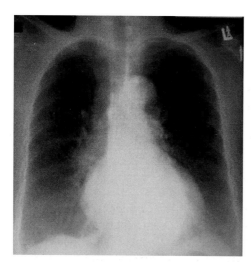

Fig. 1.38 Enlarged heart. Cardiomyopathy – note the globular appearance. The differential diagnosis included pericardial effusion.

Question 12

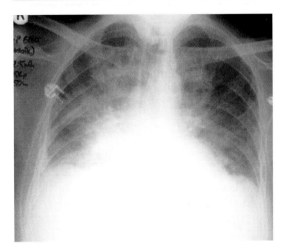

Man admitted with acute chest pain. Report this film (Fig. 1.39).

■ What is the most common cause?

Fig. 1.39 Quiz case.

Answer

Pulmonary oedema from left ventricular failure
The heart is enlarged, there is upper lobe blood diversion, septal lines (due to interstitial oedema) are present at both costophrenic angles and there is air space shadowing bilaterally in a perihilar distribution. The appearances are of pulmonary oedema from elevated pulmonary venous pressure. Ischaemic heart disease is the commonest cause.

Comment
Although in hospital practice the commonest cause of pulmonary oedema is left ventricular failure, the other causes (see Table 1.4) should also be considered if only to exclude them. Distinction can be difficult on the chest X-ray alone. In cases of elevated pulmonary venous pressure, different X-ray signs develop progressively as it rises. Clinical history, signs and further investigations all help to limit the diagnosis. Response to treatment, e.g. diuretics is helpful.

Signs of pulmonary venous hypertension
The various X-ray signs appear as progressive elevation of the venous pressure occurs (see Table 1.5). The radiological changes correlate with pulmonary capillary wedge pressure (PCWP). The X-ray changes in the lungs of patients with chronic left ventricular failure develop at PCWPs which are about 5 mmHg higher than patients with acute disease and vascular redistribution is not seen until later.

33

1

Table 1.4 Causes of pulmonary oedema

- Left ventricular failure
  - Ischaemic
  - Cardiomyopathy
- Valvular heart disease
  - Aortic/mitral
- Near drowning
- Aspiration
- ARDS (refer to Fig. 1.49)
- Altitude
- Raised intracranial pressure
- Renal failure and fluid overload

Table 1.5 Signs of pulmonary venous hypertension

1. **Vascular redistribution (PCWP 11–19 mmHg)**
   Upper lobe vessels (arteries and veins)
   Increased in diameter (greater than 3 mm in first intercostal space)
   Lower lobe vessels reduced in size

2. **Interstitial oedema (PCWP > 19 mmHg)**
   Kerley's B lines
   Bronchial cuffing

3. **Alveolar oedema (PCWP > 25 mmHg)**
   Perihilar-bat wing distribution
   Symmetrical
   Clears rapidly with diuretics

4. **Pleural effusions**

Question 13

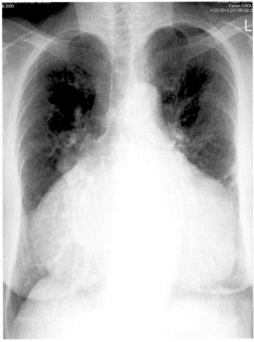

53-year-old female.
Atrial fibrillation (Fig. 1.40).

■ What is the diagnosis?

1

Fig. 1.40 Quiz case.

Answer

Mitral valve disease
The radiological features are

1. left atrial enlargement (double right heart border),

2. right ventricular enlargement,

3. posterior displacement of the oesophagus,

4. mitral valve calcification,

5. Kerley's B lines,

6. pulmonary microlithiasis (if chronic).

Question 14

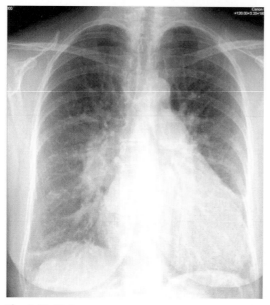

Comment (Fig. 1.41) on

1. Cardiac size.

2. Pulmonary vascularity.

3. Suggest a possible cause.

Fig. 1.41 Quiz case.

Answer

The heart is enlarged. The pulmonary trunk and the pulmonary arteries are enlarged. There is pulmonary arterial hypertension. The aortic arch is relatively small. Atrial septal defect (ASD) is the cause in this case.

Atrial septal defect

ASD causes increased pulmonary arterial flow due to blood being shunted from the left to the right atrium and, subsequently, through the pulmonary arteries and veins. This overcirculation causes pulmonary plethora making the vessels appear distended. The right atrium, right ventricle, pulmonary artery and veins become enlarged. The vessels appear crisper than pulmonary venous hypertension (due to lack of oedema) and upper lobe distension is absent. After time persistent overcirculation through the pulmonary arteries results in increased pulmonary resistance and rapid tapering of the pulmonary arteries – pruning. Reversal of the shunt can occur with time – Eisenmenger reaction. Calcification may develop in the pulmonary arteries in cases of chronic pulmonary hypertension (Table 1.6).

Table 1.6 **Causes of pulmonary hypertension**

- Chronic pulmonary venous hypertension, e.g. mitral valve disease

- Congenital heart disease with left to right shunts
  - ASD
  - VSD
  - PDA (see Figs 1.42 and 1.43)

- Pulmonary emboli

- Primary pulmonary arterial hypertension

- Chronic lung disease

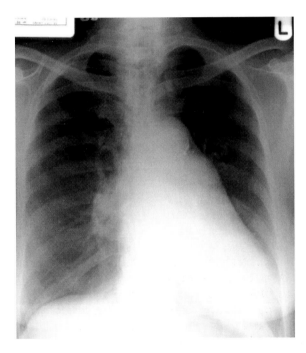

Fig. 1.42 Patent ductus arteriosus (PDA), is a cause of pulmonary hypertension – note the pulmonary artery enlargement.
A metallic coil has been placed to occlude the ductus arteriosus.

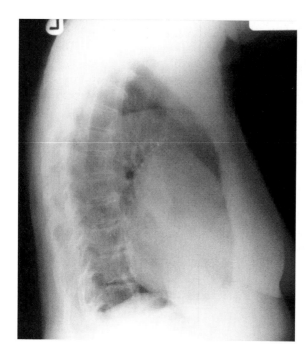

Fig. 1.43 PDA lateral projection.

Question 15

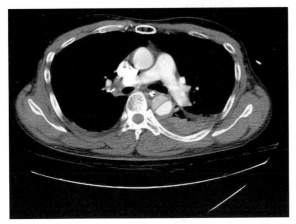

71-year-old male. Sudden onset of severe, tearing chest pain.

- What is the diagnosis (Fig. 1.44)?

Fig. 1.44 Quiz case.

Answer

Aortic dissection

The features demonstrated on the CT scan are an aortic intimal flap and a false lumen (which on higher slices starts distal to the left subclavian artery) – the features are typical of a type-B aortic dissection.

Aortic dissection has a peak incidence in the sixth to seventh decade with a male predominance. The associated risk factors are hypertension and medial degeneration. A variety of congenital diseases are associated with dissection and these include Marfan's and Ehlers–Danlos syndrome. Pregnancy and cardiac catheterisation are further risk factors.

The aorta is composed of three layers (intima, media and adventitia) and dissection is characterised by haematoma in the media of the aortic wall. The separation of the intima from the adventitia finally creates a false lumen that continues for a variable distance. If the dissection ruptures through the adventitia haemopericardium or haemothorax can result.

Stanford classification

- Type A: involving ascending aorta or arch.

- Type B: limited to descending aorta (distal to left sub-clavian).

Clinical manifestations vary depending on the site and extent of the dissection. ECG changes of myocardial infarction can be present if the coronary arteries are involved, and neurological signs may indicate haematoma or intimal flap narrowing the head and neck vessels.

Patients with Sandford type-B dissection are treated medically with management of hypertension and those with type A are treated surgically. Diagnostic imaging modalities include transthoracic and trans-oesophageal echocardiography, angiography, CT and MRI.

Question 16

34-year-old female. Taking oral contraceptive pill.
Immobilised for compound tibial fracture.
Suddenly short of breath.

■ What is the diagnosis (Fig. 1.45)?

■ What other methods of diagnostic imaging are available?

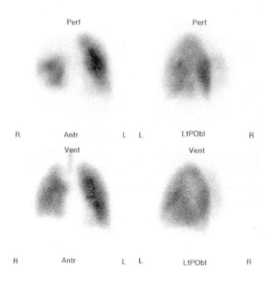

Fig. 1.45 Quiz case.

Answer

Pulmonary embolism

Pulmonary embolism (PE) is a huge problem with as many as 5% of all inpatient deaths being related to PE. Predisposing causes include bed rest, recent surgery, venous insufficiency, recent fracture and malignancy.

Major emboli usually originate in pelvic and lower leg veins although upper limb veins, cardiac chambers and central catheters are also potential sites. The clinical picture is often non-specific.

The chest X-ray is usually abnormal and signs include atelectasis, pleural effusion, elevated hemidiaphragm, prominent pulmonary artery and cardiomegaly. Focal oligaemia is uncommon and the chest X-ray is usually non-specific and, therefore, unhelpful. A rare but specific sign of PE is the Hampton's hump (Fig. 1.46). This is haemorrhagic infarction of the lung usually seen as a peripheral ill defined wedge-shaped opacity with convex borders.

Ventilation perfusion scintigraphy has been the method used in most centres to diagnose PE for some time. This involves obtaining perfusion 'Q' images of the lungs and ventilation 'V' images and comparing the two studies. Isotope labelled 'microspheres' are injected and a small proportion of these wedge in the pulmonary circulation where their position is imaged with a gamma camera. The ventilation part of the study is made during inhalation of a radioactive gas. These V/Q scans are classified as normal, high, intermediate or low probability of PE. In classic PE several large perfusion defects are identified but ventilation is normal – there is ventilation perfusion mismatch high probability of PE (see Fig. 1.45).

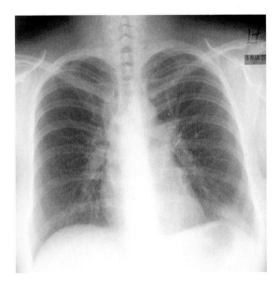

Fig. 1.46 Hampton's hump. Haemorrhagic infarction caused by PE.

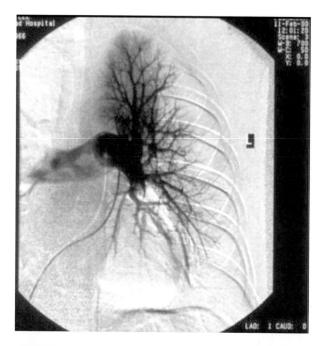

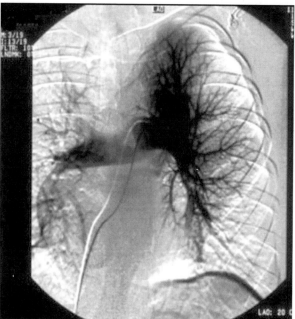

Fig. 1.47 Pulmonary arteriogram – pulmonary embolus. The catheter is seen in the left pulmonary artery. There is a substantial filling defect/clot which is reducing filling of the left lower lobe pulmonary artery and its segmental branches.

With other chest pathologies such as collapse and consolidation, both the perfusion *and* the ventilation images are abnormal – matched ventilation perfusion defects low probability of PE.

The management of patients with normal or high probability V/Q studies is straight forward, but patients with intermediate probability scans still have a 30% incidence of PE.

Pulmonary angiography (see Fig. 1.47) will demonstrate filling defects in the pulmonary circulation and is considered a reliable although invasive test for PE.

CT pulmonary angiography (see Fig. 1.48) will reliably identify clot in lobar and segmental vessels with greater than 90% sensitivity and specificity. The significance of subsegmental clots (missed on CT) is unknown. The great advantage of CT is that it will identify unsuspected pathology (e.g. lung carcinoma) which is the true cause of clinical symptoms.

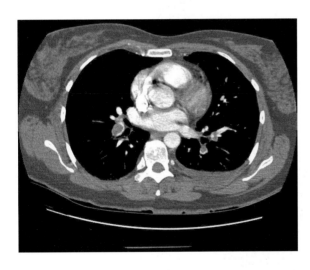

Fig. 1.48 Pulmonary embolus CT pulmonary arteriogram. Filling defects/blood clot is present in the pulmonary arteries bilaterally.

Question 17

54-year-old male.
Ventilated on the intensive care unit.

- Describe the radiological signs (Fig. 1.49).
- What is the differential diagnosis?
- How can the differential diagnosis be limited?

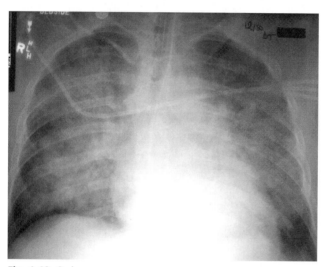

Fig. 1.49 Quiz case.

Answer

Air space shadowing: adult respiratory distress syndrome (ARDS)

The patient is clearly unwell, is ventilated and has lines including a central venous catheter (CVC) and ECG monitoring. The endotracheal tube and CVC are appropriately sited. The CVC tip should sit in the SVC and not in the right artium. In addition, there is perihilar air space shadowing involving both lungs. The differential diagnosis for such an appearance includes air space filling with infective exudate, oedema fluid, blood and malignant cells. In this situation ARDS, extensive infection or pulmonary haemorrhage seem the most likely. To limit the differential diagnosis further, more clinical information would be necessary. PCWP can be helpful. The diagnosis in the case example above was ARDS. The CT features of ARDS characteristically show dependent consolidation with more anterior ground glass shadowing (Fig. 1.50).

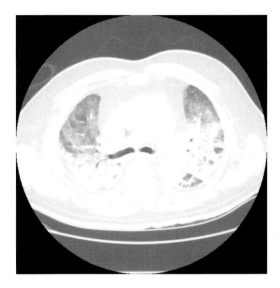

1

Fig. 1.50 CT ARDS. Dependent consolidation anterior ground glass shadowing.

Comment

On a film with diffuse increased pulmonary opacification you have to decide early on whether it is air space/consolidation or interstitial pattern shadowing. Air space shadowing has a number of characteristic features. It has poorly defined margins, a tendency to coalesce, produces air bronchograms and air alveolagrams. The causes of air space shadowing are extensive. If a chest X-ray simply shows a focal patch of consolidation and there are no further radiological clues or clinical history, it is often not possible to come to a single diagnosis.

In an examination or viva, a number of different types of air space shadowing films can be shown, e.g. ARDS with tubes and lines from ITU. Although time-consuming, it is important to check all tubes and lines for abnormal positioning. Look for rib fractures as a clue to contusion, renal dialysis double lumen lines, coronary care identification markers, etc. In these situations, it is possible to limit the differential diagnosis and then you must list the likely causes in reducing order of likelihood (Table 1.7).

1

Table 1.7 Causes of consolidation/air space shadowing

Infective exudate

Bacterial (Fig. 1.51)	*Pneumococcus, Haemophilus, Legionella, Klebsiella*
	TB (look at name)
Fungal	Histoplasmosis
Viral	Chickenpox
	Influenza
	Mycoplasma
Parasitic	Pneumocystis (although initially interstial pattern)

Pulmonary oedema

Cardiogenic	Look for ECG leads, CCU label on ID (Fig. 1.52) NB: in acute MI the heart size may be normal
Renal failure	Look for dialysis line, a double lumen central line
Neurogenic	
Noxious gas inhalation	
Narcotics	
Near drowning	
Aspiration	Look for hiatus hernia, achalasia
Altitude	
Aspirin OD	
ARDS	ITU film, lines, ECG leads, intubation
Amniotic fluid/Fat embolus	Long bone fracture

Blood

Contusion	Rib fracture, other trauma
Pulmonary haemorrhage	
Pulmonary infarct	Not strictly blood but fits best in this category

Malignant cells

Alveolar cell carcinoma (Fig. 1.53)
Lymphoma
Choriocarcinoma mets

Others

Sarcoid	
Loefflers	
BOOP (Fig. 1.54)	
PMF	
Alveolar proteinosis	
Radiation pneumonitis	
Drugs	Amiodarone produces dense consolidation

1

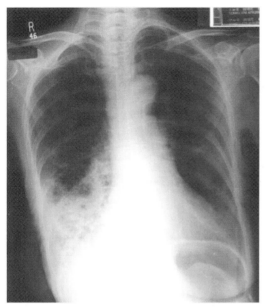

Fig. 1.51 Lobar pneumonia with air space shadowing.

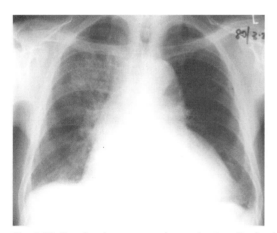

Fig. 1.52 Focal pulmonary oedema. Acute mitral valve failure. This patient was on coronary care (admitted for acute myocardial infarction), and became suddenly short of breath. The heart is enlarged and there is a patch of air space shadowing in the right mid- and upper zone. This is caused by acute mitral regurgitation in the setting of papillary muscle rupture. The regurgitant jet is directed toward the right lung.

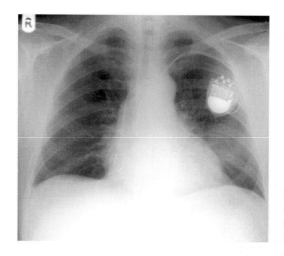

Fig. 1.53 Alveolar cell carcinoma. An area of air space shadowing is present in the left lower zone.

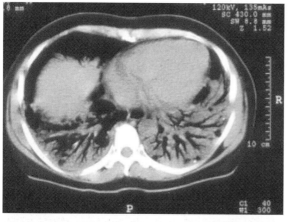

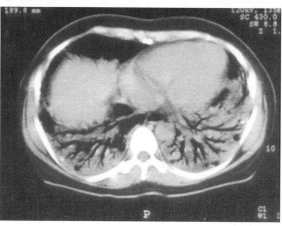

Fig. 1.54 BOOP (bronchiolitis obliterans organising pneumonia). This CT is a fine example of why consolidation/air space shadowing causes air bronchograms. On a conventional chest X-ray, air bronchograms would be seen where the air-filled bronchi are surrounded by soft tissue.

Question 18

68-year-old man.
Increasing breathlessness over past 4–5 months.
Finger clubbing. Inspiratory crackles at lung bases.

■ What is the diagnosis (Fig. 1.55)?

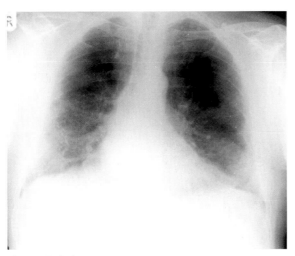

Fig. 1.55 Quiz case.

Answer

Fibrosing alveolitis
There is a fine linear and nodular pattern of increased density in both lungs predominantly in the lower zones. The heart outline is shaggy – the appearances are of an interstial lung pattern and given the clinical history would fit with fibrosing alveolitis.

Interstitial diseases
Interstitial pattern shadowing is caused by thickening of the tissue surrounding the alveoli and capillaries in the lung. Probably the most well-recognised appearance is Kerly's B lines. These are short, horizontal lines in the lung bases which reach the pleura. These not only occur in heart failure but also in lymphangitis carcinomatosa.

Various types of interstitial pattern shadowing are described and these can occur in isolation or in combination such as reticular-nodular:

■ Fine netting: reticular
■ Coarse mesh: honeycomb pattern
■ Fine lines: linear
■ Innumerable tiny nodules: nodular

Interstitial pulmonary fibrosis or fibrosing alveolitis is an idiopathic disease which causes inflammation and later lung fibrosis. Chest X-rays show an interstitial pattern which predominantly affects the bases. The lung volumes are reduced unless there is co-existing chronic obstructive pulmonary disease when lung volumes can look normal. CT or HRCT (high resolution CT) demonstrates the interstitial shadowing (Fig. 1.56) is in a peripheral distribution. Ground glass shadowing (which does not obscure pulmonary vasculature) may also be present. This can sometimes correlate with active inflammation and increased likelihood of steroid response (Table 1.8).

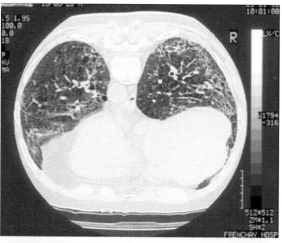

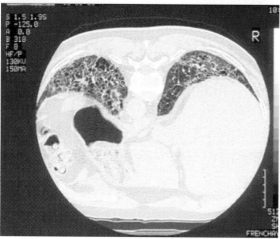

Fig. 1.56 CT fibrosing alveolitis. Peripherally distributed fibrosis and honeycombing. The patient is positioned prone as dependent fluid can cause diagnosic dilemma (particularly if the changes are less marked than this example).

Table 1.8 Causes of interstitial pattern shadowing

■ Chronic obstructive pulmonary disease (COPD)

■ Interstitial pulmonary oedema

■ Pulmonary fibrosis (Fig. 1.57)

■ Dust exposure

■ Asbestosis

■ Connective tissue diseases

■ Sarcoid

■ Drugs

■ Infection (mycoplasma, pneumocystis)

■ Lymphangitis carcinomatosa

Paediatric

■ Oxygen toxicity

■ Acute bronchiolitis (also overinflation and small patches of consolidation)

■ Cystic fibrosis (Fig. 1.58)

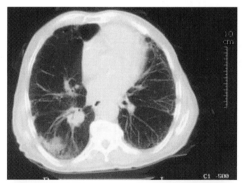

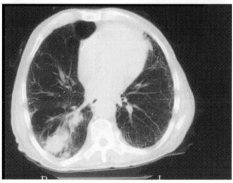

Fig. 1.57 Fibrosing alveolitis. There is peripheral fibrotic change and a mass in the right lung. The incidence of bronchial neoplasm is increased in fibrosing alveolitis.

51

1

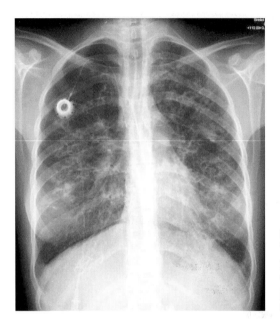

Fig. 1.58 Cystic fibrosis (CF). The widespread interstitial pattern shadowing is typical of CF. Note the right-sided portacath and a right-sided apical pneumothorax.

Question 19

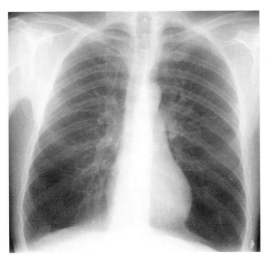

46-year-old smoker.
On surgical waiting list for
hernia surgery (Fig. 1.59).

■ What is the diagnosis?

Fig. 1.59 Quiz case.

Answer

Emphysema

There is hyperexpansion of both lungs with flattening of the diaphragms.
At the level of the diaphragm there are eight anterior ribs (normal is
six to seven). There are decreased lung markings throughout the lungs
particularly affecting the lung bases, a pattern found in alpha-1-antitrypsin
deficiency. Radiological changes of chronic bronchitis and emphysema
chronic obstructive pulmonary disease (COPD) include:

■ hyperinflation (increased retrosternal clear space on lateral film),

■ flattening of diaphragms,

■ reduced lung markings (emphysema),

■ peribronchial thickening,

■ bullae (increased risk of pneumothorax),

■ cardiac enlargement,

■ enlarged pulmonary arteries (pulmonary hypertension).

Question 20

70-year-old man. Awaiting total hip replacement. Seen in surgical pre-assessment clinic. History of cough.

■ Describe the abnormality seen on the chest X-ray (Fig. 1.60).

■ What are the most likely differential diagnoses?

■ How would you manage the patient?

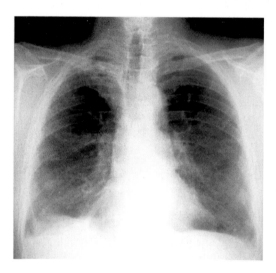

Fig. 1.60 Quiz case.

Answer

Solitary pulmonary nodule or mass

There is a solitary nodule seen in the mid-zone of the right lung.
No other pulmonary nodules or rib lesions are seen.

Nipple shadows can often cause confusion on plain films as they may resemble lung nodules. If any doubt exists then metallic skin markers should be positioned and further X-rays taken. This case example was a nipple shadow (see Fig. 1.61).

A common cause of true pulmonary nodule in a patient of this age would be bronchogenic carcinoma; metastasis, granuloma or infection are further possibilities.

Solitary pulmonary nodule

With this type of film (especially in a viva situation) you give the most likely differential diagnosis first and list the others in reducing order of probability. It is no good giving Wegeners granulomatosis as the opening differential, although possible, it is not the most likely diagnosis in a 70-year-old smoker (Table 1.9).

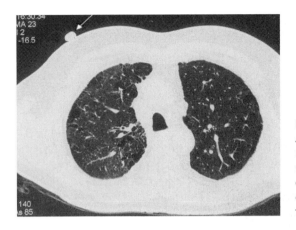

Fig. 1.61 Nipple shadow CT. Although a plain film with metallic nipple markers is usually sufficient, this CT clearly demonstrates the cause of the 'nodule' seen on the plain film.

Table 1.9 **The solitary lung mass**

Acquired

Tumour

Malignant	Bronchogenic carcinoma (look for rib mets)
Solitary metastasis	Breast (mastectomy), renal (surgical clips), sarcoma, seminoma
Lymphoma	
Benign	Carcinoid (central position)
	Hamartoma (popcorn calcification) (see Fig. 1.62)

Infection

Bacterial	Round pneumonias (children)
Parasitic	Hydatid (?name, waterlilly sign)
Fungal	Histoplasmosis

Infarction

Pulmonary	Infarct (peripheral, wedge shaped)

Vascular

Pulmonary avm	(Large feeding vessel) (see Fig. 1.63)

Granuloma

TB	(Name, satellite lesion)
Wegeners	(Old films, ?dialysis line) (Fig. 1.64)
Sarcoid	
Rheumatoid nodule	(Shoulder erosions, clavicle)

Trauma

Haematoma	(Rib fractures)

Congenital

Sequestered segment	(Usually basal)
Bronchogenic cyst	(Normally mediastinal)

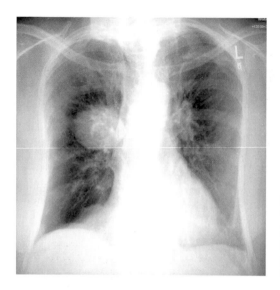

Fig. 1.62 Hamartoma. 'Popcorn' calcification is almost pathonomonic of hamartoma, usually the lesion is slow growing and about half contain fat on CT.

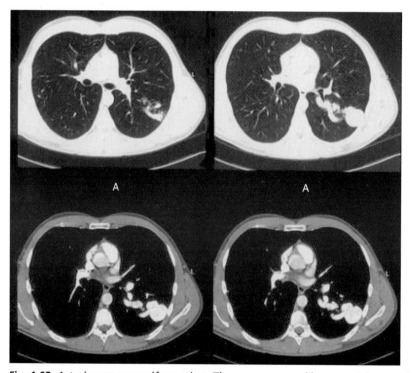

Fig. 1.63 Arterio-venous malformation. These can appear like a suspicious nodule on chest X-ray. Feeding vessels are sometimes visible on the conventional X-ray but CT with contrast enhancement will demonstrate these very elegantly.

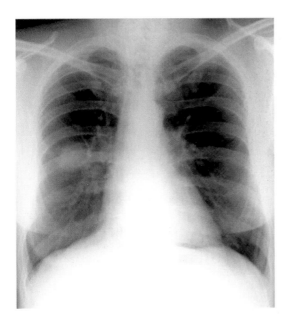

Fig. 1.64 Wegeners granulomatosis. This can appear as patchy alveolar infiltrate – either single or multiple which can also be complicated by cavitation.

You may be pressed for further causes of a solitary nodule by the examiner. This is a classic example of where to use a surgical sieve. You must try and narrow the differential by looking for any secondary signs on the film (look for the signs given in brackets).

Question 21

54-year-old male.
Chronic cough productive of sputum.
Recent fever malaise and haemoptysis.

- What is the underlying lung condition (Fig. 1.65)?

- What complication has occurred?

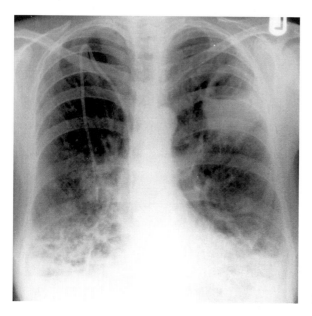

Fig. 1.65 Quiz case.

Answer

Bronchiectasis with pulmonary abscess/cavity

Causes of lung cavitation are listed in Table 1.10. In the case of lung abscesses a solid nodule is the first radiological manifestation. When the necrotic centre/pus discharges into the bronchial tree, then a fluid level and the cavity wall are often visible. In addition to pyogenic infections, a parenchymal lung cavity should raise the possibility of TB. This represents reactivation disease and classically affects the apical or posterior segments of the upper lobes. Pulmonary cavities can become complicated by empyema (Fig. 1.66).

Cavitating malignancy can appear similar to infectious cavities. These may be primary bronchogenic malignancy or metastatic disease such as head and neck squamous carcinoma. Cavitating malignancy tends to have more nodular, thicker walls (more than 15 mm) than infection (less than 5 mm).

Table 1.10 **Causes of lung cavities**

Pyogenic abscess	*Staphlococcus aureus* Beta-haemolytic streptococcus *Klebsiella* Anaerobes Septic emboli
TB	Reactivation (apical or posterior segment of upper lobes)
Parasitic infection	Echinococcus
Malignancy	Primary or metastatic (particularly squamous cell carcinoma)
Rheumatoid nodule	
Wegener's granulomatosis	
Cavitating infarct	

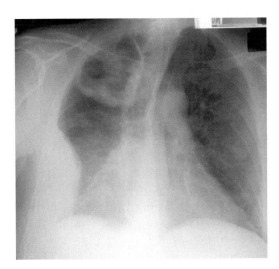

Fig. 1.66 Infective lung cavity which has been complicated by empyema.

Mimics of cavitating lesions include pneumatoceles, emphesematous bullae and cystic bronchiectasis. Pneumatoceles are thin-walled intra-parenchymal areas of air trapping which occur in the recovery phase of staphylococcal pneumonia, contusion or chronic ARDS.

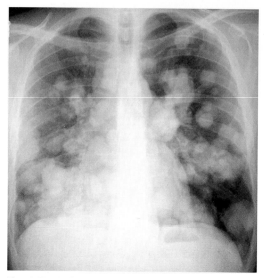

64-year-old patient.
Breathless for 2 months;
three stone weight loss.

■ What is the most likely
diagnosis (Fig. 1.67)?

Fig. 1.67 Quiz case.

Answer

Multiple pulmonary masses

There are multiple pulmonary masses of varying sizes seen in both lungs.
The commonest cause of this appearance in a patient of this age would be
multiple metastases. There are no bony lesions, no mastectomy and
no other clues to suggest a primary site. Old films would help to confirm
the nature of the nodules and rate of growth.

Comment

If pushed, this film is another situation where a surgical sieve will help to
recall causes of multiple pulmonary nodules/masses (Table 1.11).

Table 1.11 **Causes of multiple pulmonary nodules/masses**

Tumour	
Metastasis	Breast, renal, thyroid, squamous carcinoma (head and neck), gastrointestinal tumours, osteosarcoma
Lymphoma	
Infection	
Bacterial	Abscesses, *Staph. aureus, Pseudomonas*, TB
Parasitic	Hydatid
Infarction	
Multiple pulmonary infarct	
Vascular	
Pulmonary avm	
Granuloma	
Wegeners	
Rheumatoid nodule	
AIDS	
Kaposi sarcoma	
Occupation	
Caplans, PMF	
Others	
Amyloid	
Papillomatosis of the lung	

1

Question 23

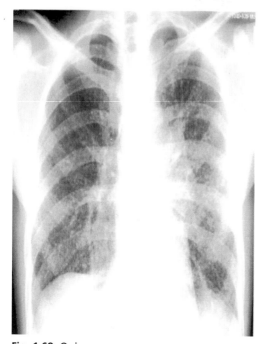

28-year-old male.
This patient is breathless febrile and unwell. He has recently arrived from Africa.

■ What is the diagnosis (Fig. 1.68)?

■ What precautions must you take with this patient?

■ If ventilation is required what further measures must be taken?

Fig. 1.68 Quiz case.

Answer

Miliary nodules

There are multiple miliary nodules in both lungs (see CT Fig. 1.69).
The patient is from Africa and is unwell making miliary TB the most likely diagnosis. Barrier nursing in isolation should be undertaken.

TB is spread by the respiratory route, so precautions must be taken to sterilise ventilation equipment following use. Disposable equipment should be used where possible and bacterial filters should be used to protect the ITU ventilator. Medical and nursing staff are at risk of infection, full face masks and eye protection should be worn during procedures involving the airway. If he was well, consider sarcoid or pneumoconiosis (old films would help in this latter differential). Any history of primary malignancy is important, thyroid malignancy, bone sarcoma and trophoblastic disease can give rise to miliary metastases. Further less common possibilities include acute extrinsic allergic alveolitis, nodular pulmonary fibrosis and histiocytosis X.

Haematogenous metastases tend to go to the bases and inhaled dusts to the apices. Densely calcified tiny nodules have a different differential diagnosis (Table 1.12).

1

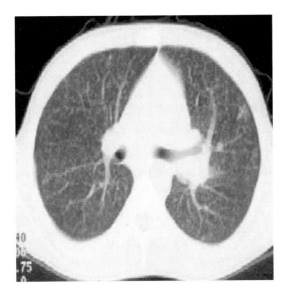

Fig. 1.69 CT miliary nodules – miliary TB. There are innumerable tiny nodules distributed throughout both lungs. The clinical setting is important in making the diagnosis as dust inhalation, granulomatous diseases, infection and metastases can give a similar appearance.

Table 1.12 **Miliary nodules**

- Miliary TB
- Sarcoid
- Dust inhalation/pneumoconiosis
- Extrinsic allergic alveolitis
- Miliary metastases: thyroid, melanoma

- Dense miliary nodules
  - Haemosiderosis
  - Silicosis
  - Stannosis
  - Chicken pox

Question 24

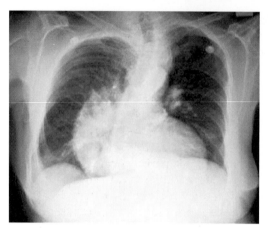

Fig. 1.70 Quiz case.

38-year-old patient. Chronic musculoskeletal deformity.

- What is this deformity (Figs 1.70 and 1.71)?

- How is it likely to affect respiratory function?

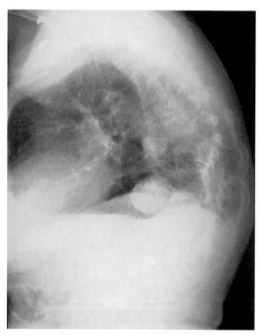

Fig. 1.71 Quiz case.

Answer

Kyphoscoliosis

Respiratory function can be affected by scoliosis. Breathing may be impaired by the chest wall deformity, resulting in alveolar hypoventilation. The chance of impairment in respiratory function is related to the maximum angle of the curvature (Cobb angle). Atelectasis and segmental collapse can occur. Chest wall deformity is seen in patients who were treated for pulmonary tuberculosis with thoracoplasty (see Fig. 1.72). Thoracoplasty was a treatment used prior to the widespread use of antibiotics. Marked chest wall deformity occurs often with considerable volume loss and sometimes with other stigmata of TB such as pleural calcification. Type II respiratory failure (hypoxia and hypercapnia) with subsequent cor pulmonale can occur. Selected patients with chronic ventilatory failure are appropriately treated with long-term domiciliary ventilation. Patients (with kyphoscoliosis and thoracoplasty) treated with non-invasive positive pressure ventilation can have improved prognosis. A nasal mask and continuous positive pressure ventilation is the usual method employed (Table 1.13).

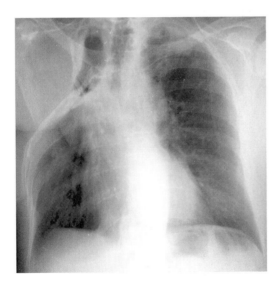

Fig. 1.72 TB thoracoplasty. Pre-antibiotic era treatment for TB.

Table 1.13 **Causes of chronic respiratory failure**

- Type I respiratory failure (hypoxia)
  - Pulmonary fibrosis
  - Pulmonary vascular disease

- Type II respiratory failure (Hypoxia and Hypercapnoea)

- Airways disease
  - Chronic obstructive pulmonary disease
  - Cystic fibrosis and bronchiectasis
  - Obstructive sleep apnoea

- Neuromuscular disorders
  - Motor neurone disease
  - Muscular dystrophy

- Thoracic cage and pleural abnormality
  - Kyphoscoliosis
  - Thoracoplasty
  - Extreme obesity

Question 25

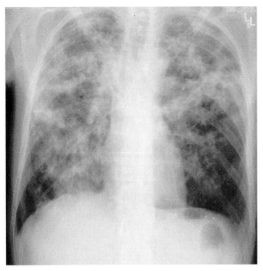

34-year-old drug addict. Homeless.
Cough and haemoptysis.
Tachypnoea, hypoxia.
You are asked to assess with view to ventilatory support.

■ What does the chest X-ray (Fig. 1.73) show?

■ What risk factors should be considered?

Fig. 1.73 Quiz case.

Answer

Pulmonary tuberculosis

There are confluent ill-defined areas of consolidation in the mid- and upper zones of both lungs. Given the appearance and distribution of the changes, pulmonary TB has to be a primary consideration. Altered immunity from HIV should be considered (Table 1.14).

Table 1.14 **Chest X-ray manifestations of TB**

■ Primary pulmonary TB
- Air space consolidation 1–7 cm diameter
- Lymphadenopathy: hilar, paratracheal
- Pleural effusion
- Segmental consolidation
- Cavitation
- Calcified ghon focus
- Calcified lymph nodes

■ Post-primary TB (reactivation or initial infection or infection post-BCG)
- Apical and posterior segments of upper lobes
- Chronic patchy ill-defined areas of opacification
- Cavitation may colonise with *Aspergillus*
- Bronchiectasis
- Upper lobe fibrosis (see Fig. 1.74)

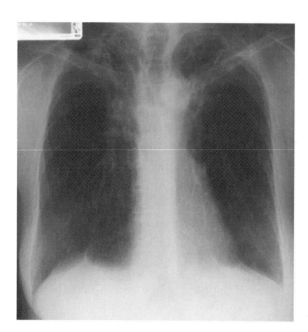

Fig. 1.74 TB upper lobe fibrosis. There is linear shadowing and volume loss in both upper zones with elevation of both hila.

Question 26

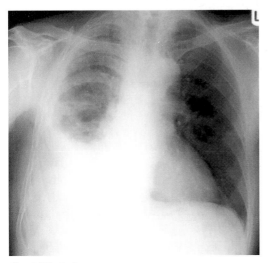

68-year-old electrician. 6 months of worsening chest pain.

- What is the diagnosis (Figs 1.75 and 1.76)?

- What further question will help make a diagnosis?

- Describe the procedure to confirm the diagnosis.

Fig. 1.75 Quiz case.

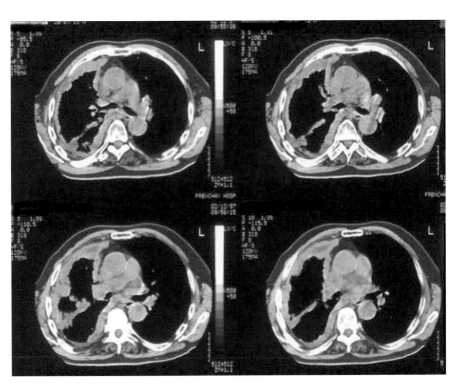

Fig. 1.76 Quiz case.

Answer

Mesothelioma

Electricians in the past were frequently exposed to asbestos and this is a crucial question to ask in the clinical history.

Pleural biopsy will confirm the diagnosis. This has traditionally been carried out blind, i.e. without image guidance. The procedure is carried out with the patient seated comfortably and leaning forward with the posterior of the chest wall exposed. Using the chest X-ray for localisation, under sterile conditions, the superficial tissues are infiltrated with local anaesthetic at a suitable rib interspace. A biopsy needle is inserted adjacent to the superior rib border (to avoid the neurovascular bundle) and the pleural biopsy taken. Ultrasound can be used to identify pleural thickening, and thereby guide biopsy and target potentially pathological areas.

Malignant mesothelioma is often related to previous asbestos exposure with a lag period of up to 30 years or more. It usually presents as a multilobulated pleural mass encircling the lung. It involves the mediastinal pleural reflections and often extends into the lung fissures or out to the chest wall, particularly, along a biopsy track. Pericardial involvement or diaphragmatic invasion can occur. Pleural effusions are common and these may be loculated. Other manifestations of asbestos exposure include pleural calcification, folded lung (see Fig. 1.77) (which may be mistaken for a malignant mass) and asbestosis.

Causes of pleural malignancy

- Bronchial adenocarcinoma.

- Breast carcinoma.

- Malignant thymoma.

- Subpleural lymphoma.

- Malignant mesothelioma.

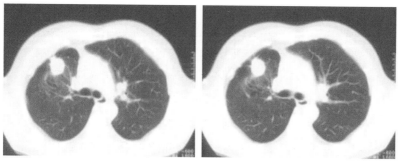

Fig. 1.77 Asbestos lung disease rounded atelectasis. Also called Folded lung, is frequently adjacent to a site of pleural thickening – vessels normally converge towards it in a characteristic way.

Question 27

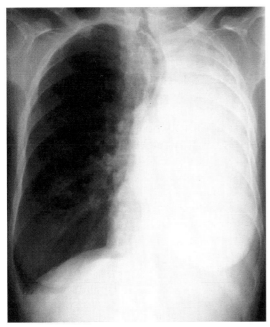

76-year-old man.
Life-long smoker.
Cough and haemoptysis.

■ What is the diagnosis
(Fig. 1.78)?

1

Fig. 1.78 Quiz case.

Answer

Collapse of the left lung

There is almost total collapse of the left lung, due to an underlying
bronchogenic malignancy. Note the volume loss with shift of
the mediastinum to the affected side (Table 1.15).

Table 1.15 **Causes of opaque hemithorax**

■ *Lung collapse*: volume loss, mediastinal shift towards affected side

■ *Pleural fluid*: transudate/exudate; empyema; haemothorax; chylothorax

■ *Pneumonectomy*: look for surgical clips and thoracotomy

■ *Tumour*: fibrous tumour of pleura; pleural metastases; mesothelioma

■ *Extensive consolidation*: pneumonia; pulmonary oedema; obstructing
neoplasm

■ *Lung agenesis*

Question 28

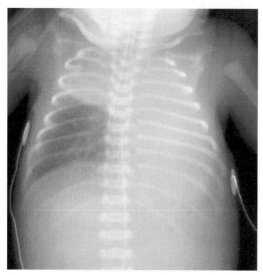

2-week-old neonate.

■ What does the chest X-ray (Fig. 1.79) demonstrate?

Fig. 1.79 Quiz case.

Answer

Malpositioned endotracheal tube

If an endotracheal tube is positioned incorrectly within the major airways, then lobar collapse can follow in the under ventilated lobes. In this example, the endotracheal tube has been passed along the right main bronchus distal to the origin of the right upper lobe bronchus with subsequent collapse of the right upper lobe and the left lung.

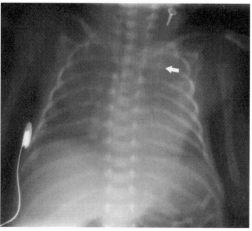

Fig. 1.80 The left-sided central venous line is too lateral on the check X-ray.

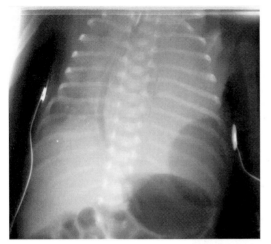

Fig. 1.81 On the basis of the X-ray in Fig. 1.17 the central venous line was used for parenteral nutrition. There is now a large left-sided pleural fluid collection – the line tip was clearly positioned in the pleural space.

In Figs 1.80 and 1.81 a left-sided central line has been placed in the pleural space (the line appears too lateral) and intravenous nutrition has been infiltrated into the pleural cavity compressing the left lung and the mediastinum.

Question 29

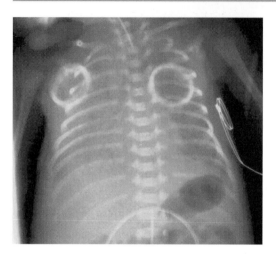

18-hour-old male neonate. Tachypnoea, sternal and intercostal rescession.

■ What does the chest X-ray (Fig. 1.82) show?

Fig. 1.82 Quiz case.

Answer

Respiratory distress syndrome

This is the most common, serious respiratory disorder in neonates (Table 1.16). It is caused by lack of surfactant (normally produced by type II pneumocytes). It is a condition usually associated with prematurity but may also occur in term neonates of diabetic mothers or following birth asphyxia. The normal time of onset is at 18–24 hours of life. The radiological signs are initially of under-inflated lungs which have a granular appearance. With worsening disease air bronchograms become more prominent and this can partially obscure the mediastinal contours. Very premature babies and those with bad respiratory distress syndrome (RDS) are treated with surfactant (administered via an endotracheal tube) which usually produces a marked improvement in their condition.

Table 1.16 Possible causes of respiratory distress in a neonate

---

■ Respiratory distress syndrome

■ Transient tachypnoea of the newborn

■ Aspiration

■ Pneumothorax

■ Diaphragmatic hernia

■ Pneumonia

■ Congenital heart disease

Complications of respiratory distress

Most of the complications are secondary to mechanical ventilation.
Small airway rupture can lead to air tracking into the pleural space –
pneumothorax or the mediastinum – pneumomediastinum.

Pneumomediastinum usually produces a sharp clearly defined lucency
adjacent to each side of the mediastinum. The mediastinal borders are
usually of increased sharpness as they become outlined by air rather than
lung parenchyma (see Fig. 1.83). A horizontal beam lateral radiograph will
confirm the location of the air. The lungs are poorly compliant in RDS,
so do not collapse. The air can often be seen outlining the thymus as well
as the other mediastinal structures (see Fig. 1.84).

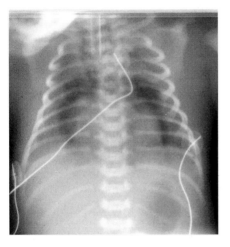

Fig. 1.83 Pneumomediastinum.
Air is present in the anterior
mediastinum outlining the heart.

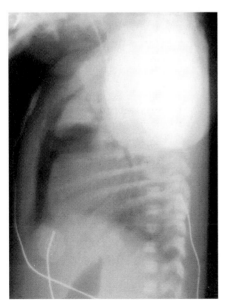

Fig. 1.84 Neonatal pneumomediastinum
lateral projection. The patient is
positioned supine and a shoot through
lateral projection has been performed.
This is outlining the thymus and other
mediastinal structures.

Question 30

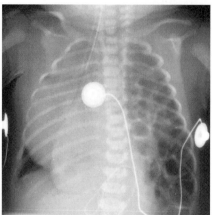

1-day-old infant with respiratory difficulties.

■ What does the X-ray (Fig. 1.85) show?

Fig. 1.85 Quiz case.

Answer

Diaphragmatic hernia
There are multiple loops of bowel within the chest causing marked shift of mediastinal structures to the opposite side. The loops of bowel in the chest are clearly continuous with those in the abdomen.

Most diaphragmatic hernias are symptomatic shortly after birth, they are more commonly left sided. The abdominal contents occupy the chest cavity in utero so both lungs (particularly on the side of the hernia) are hypoplastic. There is a significant mortality following successful surgical repair (see Table 1.16).

2

Imaging the abdomen

Plain abdominal X-rays

A systematic approach to plain abdominal X-rays will help to avoid errors in interpretation. The standard abdominal views are erect and supine AP views. Abdominal X-ray interpretation depends upon the assessment of the bowel gas pattern, solid organ outlines, a search for abnormal calcification and a review of the skeleton. A search should be made for extraluminal gas.

Bowel gas pattern

Distinguishing large from small bowel may be difficult. The presence of solid faeces, distribution, calibre and mucosal pattern of the bowel helps in deciding whether a particular loop of bowel is stomach, small intestine or colon. The presence of solid faeces indicates large bowel which may also be recognised by the incomplete haustral band crossing the colonic gas shadow. Haustra are usually present in the ascending and transverse colon but may be absent from the splenic flexure and descending colon.

The valvulae conniventes of the small bowel are closer together and cross the width of the bowel. The distal ileum when dilated can appear smooth which makes differentiation more difficult. Small bowel when obstructed is generally centrally positioned with numerous loops of tighter curvature than large bowel.

Maximum small bowel calibre is 3.5 cm in the jejunum and 2.5 cm in the ileum. Maximum calibre of the transverse colon on plain films is taken to be 5.5 cm in diameter and the maximal caecal diameter 9 cm.

Solid organs

The liver edge, renal outlines and splenic tip may all be demonstrated. The liver is seen in the right upper quadrant and extends downwards a variable distance. The tip of the right lobe may be seen extending below the right kidney – a normal variant called a Reidl's lobe. The spleen may be visualised (especially in slim individuals) even when of normal size. It enlarges inferiorly and towards the left lower quadrant. It is often possible to identify both kidneys and the psoas shadows within the retro-peritoneum. Soft tissue masses or abscess can sometimes be identified on plain films. An abscess generally has a rather heterogenous density due to the presence of gas and necrotic tissue. Mass lesions are of soft tissue density and will displace bowel gas shadows.

Calcification

Calcification should be identified and anatomically located. In some locations (such as vascular calcification) it is common and benign. Vascular calcification may be seen within the aorta, splenic artery in the left upper quadrant or in the pelvis. Calcified renal tract stones should be looked for around the renal outlines and down the line of the ureters. More rarely calcified gallstones are seen in the right upper quadrant or a calcified (porcelain) gall bladder. A calcified pancreas is diagnostic of chronic pancreatitis. Other causes of pelvic calcification include phleboliths, calcified fibroids and rarely calcification in ovarian teratodermoids. The latter may also contain teeth and hair. See normal abdominal X-ray case (see Fig. 2.1).

A careful methodical examination of all the structures of the plain abdominal film will help to avoid errors in diagnosis. The cases below have been specifically chosen to demonstrate the more commonly encountered pathologies in anaesthetic practice, the FRCA examination, and in those patients admitted to intensive care units.

2

Case illustrations: plain films and CT

Question 1

■ Name the normal structures labelled on the abdominal X-ray (Fig. 2.1).

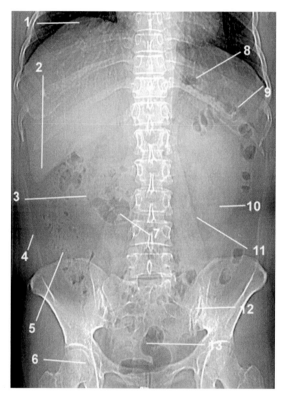

Fig. 2.1 Quiz case.

Answer

1. Right hemidiaphragm

2. Liver outline

3. Right kidney

4. Peritoneal fat line

5. Ascending colon

6. Right hip

7. Small bowel gas shadow

8. Stomach gas bubble

9. Splenic flexure

10. Lower pole of left kidney

11. Left psoas shadow

12. Left sacro-iliac joint

13. Sigmoid colon

Question 2

- Name the structures on this abdominal CT (Figs 2.2–2.5).

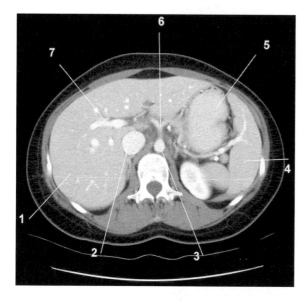

Fig. 2.2 Quiz case.

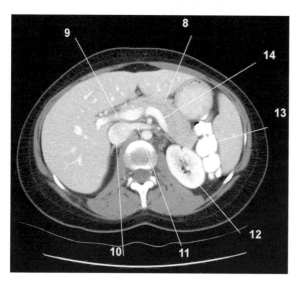

Fig. 2.3 Quiz case.

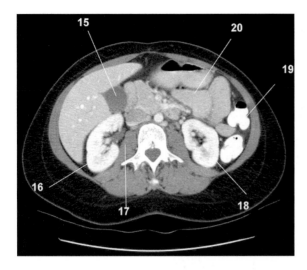

Fig. 2.4 Quiz case.

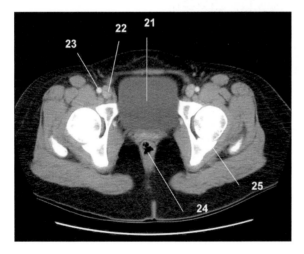

Fig. 2.5 Quiz case.

Answer

1. Right lobe of liver

2. IVC

3. Aorta

4. Spleen

5. Stomach

6. Coeliac axis

7. Right portal vein

8. Pancreas

9. Main portal vein

10. IVC

11. Left renal vein

12. Left kidney

13. Colon

14. Splenic vein

15. Gall bladder

16. Right kidney

17. Psoas

18. Left kidney

19. Colon

20. Small bowel

21. Bladder

22. Femoral vein

23. Femoral artery

24. Rectum

25. Left femoral head

Question 3

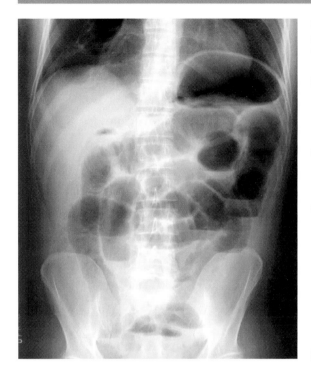

62-year-old patient. Colicky abdominal pain. Tinkling bowel sounds.

- In what position were the films (Figs 2.6 and 2.7) taken?

- Describe the abnormality on the abdominal X-ray.

- What is the management?

Fig. 2.6 Quiz case.

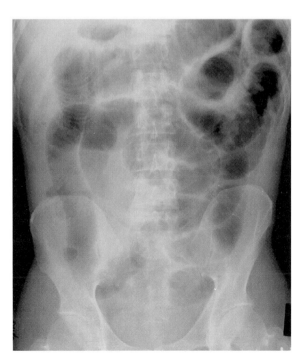

Fig. 2.7 Quiz case.

Answer

Small bowel obstruction
The films were taken erect (Fig. 2.6) and supine (Fig. 2.7).

The erect X-ray shows multiple dilated gas-filled loops of bowel with several air–fluid levels. The supine film shows multiple tightly coiled loops of centrally positioned small bowel. Gas bubbles are seen trapped against the anterior mucosal surface. The appearances are of small bowel obstruction. Referral should be made to a surgical firm. Dehydration and electrolyte imbalance should be corrected and a nasogastric tube should be passed.

Comment
Mechanical small bowel obstruction (SBO) characteristically has multiple loops of dilated, centrally positioned bowel. There are frequently numerous loops of tight curvature. These are clearly seen when gas filled, but can be very much more subtle should they be fluid filled. An erect film demonstrates multiple air–fluid levels. If loops are predominantly fluid filled then only a few scattered gas bubbles may be seen trapped against the mucosal surface. This is known as the 'string of beads' sign and is a useful sign in confirming SBO in the otherwise gasless abdominal radiograph. A paucity of large bowel gas can be a helpful sign.

Although SBO usually occurs due to post-surgical adhesions or inguinal hernia, other aetiologies will give similar appearances and these cannot be easily differentiated on the plain AXR. In cases of SBO, the hernial orifices should be scrutinised for incarcerated bowel. Gallstone ileus is a rare cause of SBO which can give a classical appearance on AXR. This occurs when a large gallstone (over 2.5 cm) passes from the gall bladder into the small bowel. If the stone is calcified then it may be seen on the abdominal film (see Fig. 2.8). This is usually identified in the right iliac fossa where it impacts in the terminal ileum commonly 60 cm proximal (narrowest part of the small bowel) to the ileo-caecal valve causing SBO. It can be symptomatic when more proximal. Chronic gall bladder inflammation leads to cholecysto-duodenal fistula and stone passage into the duodenum. Stone passage allows reflux of gas into the biliary tree giving a branching gas pattern projected over the right upper quadrant (see Fig. 2.9). At laparotomy the stone containing loop of small bowel is isolated and attempts to crush the stone can be made. If this fails the small bowel is opened proximal to the stone which is milked out.

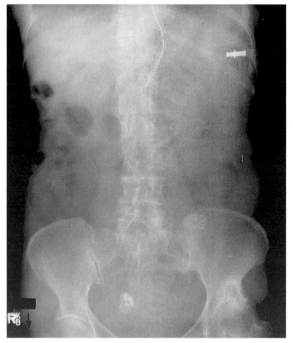

Fig. 2.8 Plain film gallstone ileus. The impacted gallstone is seen projected over the left sacro-iliac joint. A gas-filled loop of small bowel is present in the left upper quadrant. Faint branching gas shadow in the right upper quadrant. Note also the calcified pelvic fibroid.

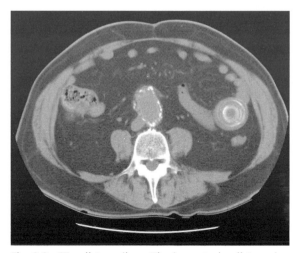

Fig. 2.9. CT gallstone ileus. The impacted gallstone is seen in the lumen of the ileum in the left flank.

87

Question 4

64-year-old patient.

This patient has a history of diabetes and had reconstructive vascular surgery for peripheral vascular disease 8 days ago. He received intravenous broad spectrum antibiotics for a surgical wound infection and now has bloody diarrhoea.

- What are the radiological signs (Fig. 2.10)?

- What is the diagnosis?

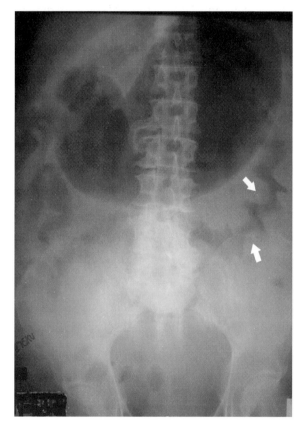

Fig. 2.10 Quiz case.

Answer

This case demonstrates colonic wall thickening, thumb printing and a distended stomach. The diagnosis is pseudomembranous colitis and diabetic gastroparesis.

Pseudomembranous colitis

In general, the radiological findings are adynamic ileus with moderate gaseous distension of the small and large bowel. The haustral folds are frequently shaggy and irregular and 'thumbprinting' is often identified particularly in the transverse colon (as in Fig. 2.10). Diffuse colonic thickening can be identified on CT. Pseudomembranous colitis is caused by an overgrowth of the commensal anaerobe *Clostridium difficile*. Commonly it is a complication of antibiotic therapy particularly ampicillin, amoxycillin, clindamycin and the cephalosporins. Antibiotic disturbance of the normal gut flora appears to allow overgrowth of toxigenic strains of *C. difficile*. The clinical and pathological effects are the result of toxin production. Further predisposing causes include bowel obstruction and co-existent debilitating disease, e.g. leukaemia. The clinical picture is of profuse diarrhoea, abdominal cramps and tenderness. A yellow exudative pseudomembrane, haemorrhagic areas and mucosal ulcers are seen on colonoscopy.

Diabetic gastroparesis is a recognised complication of diabetes mellitus when there is gastric retention in the absence of mechanical obstruction. This can be life threatening. The stomach should be decompressed and emptied with a nasogastric tube. Other causes include electrolyte imbalances (diabetic ketoacidosis), drugs, peritonitis and abdominal trauma.

2

Question 5

86-year-old female.
The patient has had several episodes of abdominal pain and distension.
She is now vomiting.

■ What is the diagnosis (Fig. 2.11)?

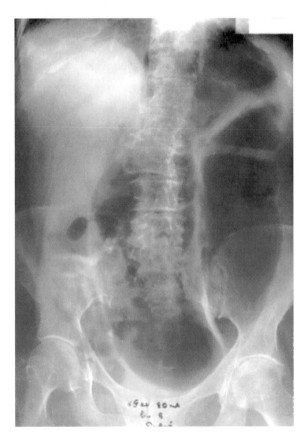

Fig. 2.11 Quiz case.

Answer

Sigmoid volvulus
This is a rotation of the gut about its own mesenteric axis, which produces complete intestinal obstruction. It is most commonly seen in the elderly or those with psychiatric disorders taking medication. Venous congestion leading to infarction can occur. On the plain abdominal film a hugely dilated loop of bowel is seen extending from the pelvis. The inverted 'U' loop is commonly devoid of haustra and is seen to extend as far as the liver in the right upper quadrant, and to the 10th thoracic vertebra superiorly. The inferior convergance of the two limbs of the loop is often

left sided. There may be some secondary loops of dilated large bowel associated with these appearances. Sigmoidoscopy can be both diagnostic and therapeutic by releasing flatus. Approximately half of patients have a further episode of volvulus within 2 years. In caecal volvulus, the caecum is seen to revolve around its axis to lie across the midline in the upper/central abdomen Fig. 2.12.

Large bowel obstruction gives rise to distention of the large bowel down to the level of obstruction sometimes with accompanying small bowel dilation. The commonest cause is colonic carcinoma. Other causes include volvulus, intussusception or extrinsic compression.

In paralytic ileus both the large and small bowel can become dilated which can extend down into the sigmoid colon and rectum (see Fig. 2.13). Differentiation from low large bowel obstruction may be difficult.

2

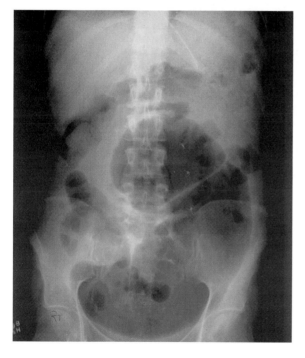

Fig. 2.12 Caecal volvulus.

2

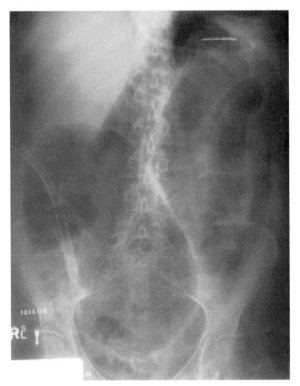

Fig. 2.13 Pseudo-obstruction. This can be difficult to distinguish from distal large bowel obstruction. Large and small bowel distension is usually present with reduced small bowel distension on serial films. If concern persists an instant enema can be performed.

Question 6

51-year-old patient.
Recurrent rectal bleeding, admitted with acute abdominal pain.

■ What is the diagnosis?

■ What are the radiological features (Fig. 2.14)?

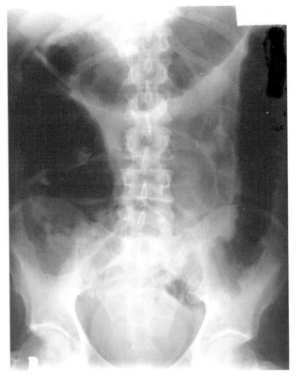

Fig. 2.14 Quiz case.

Answer

Pan colitis and perforation

The whole of the colon is distended. There is thickening of the mucosa which is oedematous. In the centre of the film there are several dilated loops of small bowel and their inner and outer walls are both visible. This latter feature indicates free gas within the peritoneal cavity.

The appearances of the bowel are characteristic of a pan colitis (affecting the whole colon) typical of ulcerative colitis. The bowel has clearly perforated. The term megacolon is frequently applied in cases of transmural fulminant colitis when the bowel looses motor tone and dilates to a transverse diameter of greater than 5.5 cm. The term *toxic* megacolon should be reserved for cases of dilatation with systemic toxicity, abnormal clinical signs (peritonism, fever) and abnormal laboratory indices (raised inflammatory markers, leukocytosis and left shift). The clinical setting is usually accompanied by profuse bloody diarrhoea. Mortality is up to 20%, barium enema is contraindicated. Ulcerative colitis is the commonest cause but others include Crohn's disease, amoebiasis, *Salmonella*, pseudomembranous and ischaemic colitis.

Extraluminal gas

Normally bowel gas is only present within the bowel lumen. This results in a clear image of the inner margin of the bowel on the abdominal X-ray. This is due to the air–mucosa interface which has different densities. The outer margin, however, is not clearly seen since the serosal surfaces merge with other adjacent bowel wall loops of similar density. However, free intra-peritoneal gas will also clearly outline the outer serosal margin of the bowel. The bowel wall thus appears as a thin 'pencilled' line with gas on either side. This appearance is known as Rigler's sign. Gas may be visible under the hemidiaphragms on an erect chest or abdominal film (Fig. 2.15).

Free gas may be seen after bowel perforation or following laparotomy. In adults, post-laparotomy pneumoperitoneum persists for up to 7 days but is absorbed very much more quickly in children, usually by 24 hours.

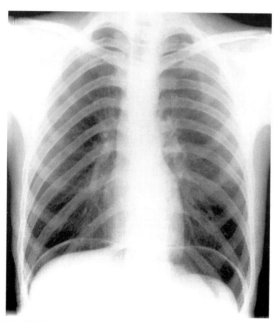

Fig. 2.15 Erect chest X-ray. Pneumoperitoneum – air under the diaphragms.

Question 7

46-year-old male.
This patient has presented with acute right iliac fossa pain.
You have been asked to assess him prior to exploratory laparotomy.

- What is the X-ray (Fig. 2.16) abnormality?

- What is the likely diagnosis?

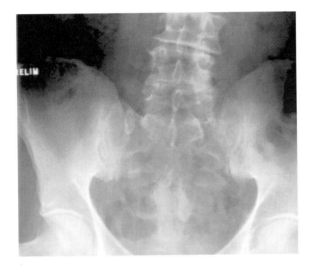

Fig. 2.16 Quiz case.

Answer

There is an oval opacity overlying the right sacral ala. The appearances are typical of a faecolith or appendolith. This calcified faecal material can occur in the appendix or a large bowel diverticulum. In conjunction with right iliac fossa pain, appendicitis is the most likely diagnosis. Ultrasound has high specificity in diagnosing appendicitis but poor sensitivity (see Fig. 2.17).

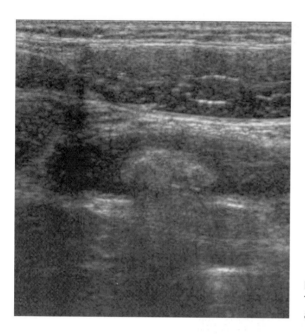

Fig. 2.17 US appendicitis. The echogenic structure is an appendicolith.

Abnormal calcification can be used to make a diagnosis in the following conditions:

- calcified aortic aneurysm;
- calcified gallstones;
- renal/ureteric stones;
- pancreas: chronic pancreatitis (Fig. 2.40);
- appendolith: appendicitis;
- liver calcification: granuloma, old abscess, some metastases;
- uterine fibroids.

Question 8

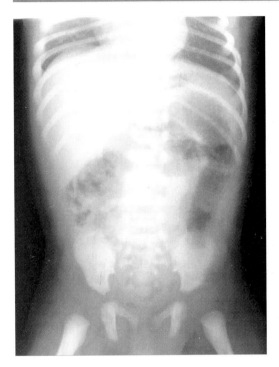

14-day-old male child.

- What is the diagnosis (Fig. 2.18)?

- What are the common associations?

- What co-existent respiratory problems are frequently encountered?

2

Fig. 2.18 Quiz case.

Answer

Necrotising enterocolitis

Gas can be seen in the wall of a distended loop of bowel (probably the transverse and descending colon). It is difficult to differentiate large from small bowel in the neonate based on bowel distribution alone. The abdomen is rather featureless elsewhere.

Other recognised radiological signs of necrotising enterocolitis (NEC) include small and large bowel dilation, a *bubbly* appearance to the bowel, gas in the portal venous system and bowel perforation. NEC most commonly (but not exclusively) affects premature neonates. Barium enema is contraindicated. In adults, gas in the bowel wall often indicates bowel infarction and has a poor prognosis. It should not be confused with pneumatosis cystoides intestinalis.

Associations of NEC:

- prematurity,

- Hirschsprung's disease,

- bowel obstruction (e.g. meconium ileus or atresia).

It is frequently co-existent with respiratory problems of the ventilated neonate such as hyaline membrane disease.

Question 9

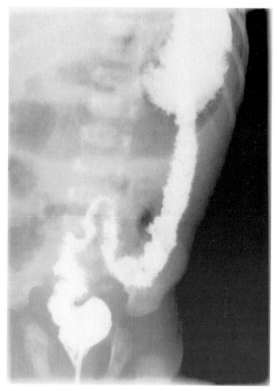

Aged 5 weeks.
History of infrequent stools (Fig. 2.19).
Abdominal distension.

- What is the examination?

- What are the important radiological features and the diagnosis?

Fig. 2.19 Quiz case.

Answer

Hirschprung's disease – barium enema

Hirschprung's disease is caused by failure of development of ganglion cells. The disease starts at the anus and a variable amount of bowel is affected proximally. Presentation can be with neonatal bowel obstruction or constipation in later life. The aganglionic segment does not transmit peristalsis so the proximal bowel dilates and the affected segment appears normal or small calibre. In the case example, there is a transition zone with dilated proximal bowel and a normal/small calibre aganglionic bowel segment. A well-recognised complication (present in the example above) is necrotising enterocolitis.

Question 10

Age 2.
This child presented with abdominal pain, and blood stained mucus PR.

■ What do the abdominal film and the ultrasound (US)
  (Figs 2.20 and 2.21) show?

■ What would you request next?

■ What precautions are necessary?

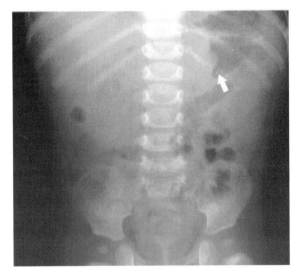

Fig. 2.20 Quiz case.

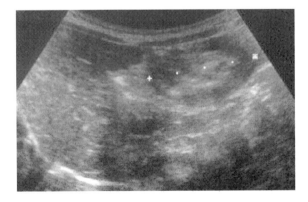

Fig. 2.21 Quiz case.

Answer

Intussusception

·The abdominal film demonstrates a soft tissue mass in the left upper quadrant in the region of the transverse colon. This is clearly outlined on one side by gas in the colon distal to it. This is the lead point of an intussusception – the clinical history is extremely suggestive in a child of this age. The ultrasound (US) confirms a mass which is characteristic of an intussusception.

Air enema/pneumatic reduction is the preferred initial method of treatment. This requires fluid resuscitation and IV antibiotics prior to the procedure. This should only be carried out in a centre with paediatric surgical cover. The procedure fails in a proportion of cases and open surgical reduction may be necessary. Pneumoperitoneum, peritonitis and hypovolaemic shock are contraindications to the technique. A large bore Foley catheter is inserted into the rectum and the buttocks are taped together. Air is insufflated using a pump with a pressure gauge that has a valve mechanism to prevent excessive pressures. The lead point of the intussusception can be followed fluoroscopically and usually reduces fairly easily (success rate is up to 90%) but there may be some hold up at the ileo-caecal valve level. When the intussusception reduces, the small bowel can be seen to suddenly fill with a puff of gas. Bowel perforation is a potential complication and this may splint the diaphragm compromising respiration. A large bore needle should be kept to hand and used to decompress a pneumoperitoneum. Incomplete reduction and recurrence in up to 10% are further complications.

2

Question 11

28-year-old female.
Dysphagia, chest pains and choking episodes.

■ What is the diagnosis (Fig. 2.22)?

■ What is the importance of this condition in anaesthetic practice?

2

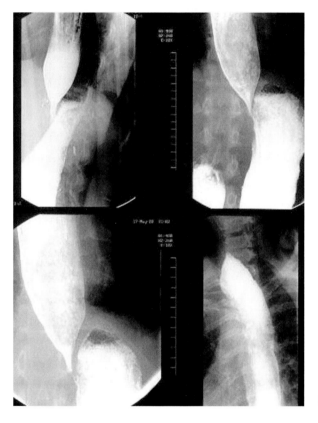

Fig. 2.22 Quiz case.

Answer

Achalasia

This is a condition of middle age caused by a reduced number of ganglion cells in the myenteric pexus. There is failure of relaxation of the lower oesophageal sphincter in response to swallowing. There is absence of peristalsis in the mid- and lower oesophagus which dilates to produce a megaoesophagus. Symptoms include dysphagia, weight loss, regurgitation and chest pain. Aspiration can occur. Sometimes, the chest X-ray is diagnostic and an air–fluid level can be seen in a dilated oesophagus. On barium examination, there is a characteristic bird beak deformity at

101

the gastro-oesophageal junction. Manometry will demonstrate an absent primary peristaltic wave and tertiary contractions.

The differential diagnosis includes infiltrating carcinoma, scleroderma and Chagas' disease.

The aim of treatment is to reduce the pressure of the lower oesophageal sphincter. Medical therapies include long-acting nitrates or calcium channel blockers. Further options include injection with botulinum toxin, balloon dilation (which may be repeated if necessary) and surgery – oesophagomyotomy which can be performed laparoscopically.

Patients are at risk of aspiration and a rapid sequence induction with cricoid pressure and endotracheal intubation must be performed if the patient requires general anaesthesia.

Question 12

Man aged 78.
Life-long smoker. Dysphagia for solids and liquids.

- What are the radiological features (Fig. 2.23)?

- What is the diagnosis?

- What are the implications for anaesthesia?

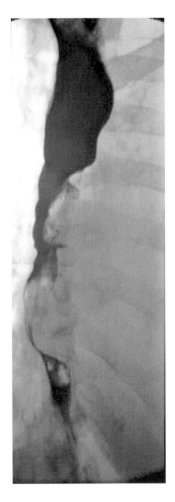

Fig. 2.23 Quiz case.

Answer

Malignant oesophageal stricture

There is a long irregular stricture affecting the mid- and lower oesophagus. The pattern of obstruction is in keeping with an extrinsic infiltrating mass. On careful inspection, it is clear that the density of the left lung is increased. The left lung has collapsed due to a mass at the hilum/mediastinum. The diagnosis is carcinoma of the left lower lobe bronchus with an associated mediastinal mass. There is extrinsic compression and invasion of the oesophagus where the mass is invading the mediastinum. The patient is not ventilating the left lung.

Surgery would be a major undertaking. The patient requires careful pre-operative assessment with careful consideration of his cardiovascular and respiratory state, and his ability to survive the procedure, before surgery is booked.

If surgery is undertaken, one-lung ventilation after placement of a double lumen tube, would facilitate surgical access. Invasive monitoring and post-operative ITU care would be required.

Question 13

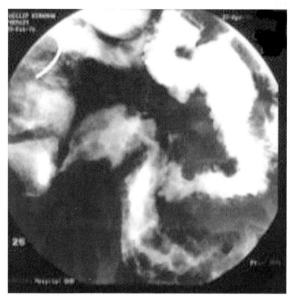

Age 34.
Recurrent episodes of right lower quadrant abdominal pain.

■ What is this examination?

■ What are the radiological features (Fig. 2.24)?

■ What is the diagnosis?

2

Fig. 2.24 Quiz case.

Answer

Crohn's disease

This is one of the images taken during a barium follow-through examination. The small bowel can be examined using a barium follow-through technique or by intubating the proximal jejunum and injecting barium – small bowel enema/enteroclysis. A number of abdominal films are taken (in the prone position to separate the small bowel loops) to examine the small bowel as the barium passes to the colon. Further views are taken of the terminal ileum as this is an area particularly affected by Crohn's disease. The case example demonstrates a thickened, nodular (cobblestone-like appearance) of the terminal ileum mucosa – typical of Crohn's disease.

Asymmetry, skip lesions, deep ulcers (see Fig. 2.25) and fistula formation are the hallmark of Crohn's disease, where as ulcerative colitis is characterised by a symmetrical disease in continuity, granular mucosa (see Figs 2.26 and 2.27), superficial ulcers and rectal involvement. In late stage, there may be inflammatory polypoid changes, narrowing and shortening of the colon. In ulcerative colitis (Fig. 2.28), the ileo-caecal valve is gaping (Table 2.1).

2

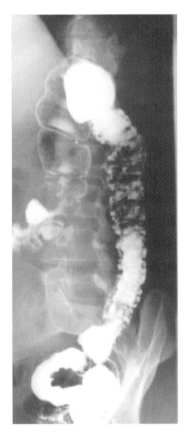

Fig. 2.25 Crohn's colon. The double contrast (air and barium) barium enema shows deep ulcers in the descending colon and the sigmoid.

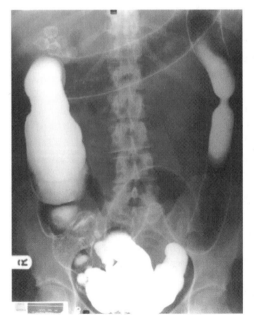

Fig. 2.26 Ulcerative colitis. The entire colon is affected, there are reduced haustral markings and the mucosa is abnormal with a fine mucosal granularity.

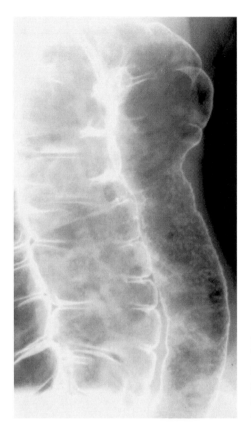

Fig. 2.27 Ulcerative colitis. The descending colon (sigmoid and rectum are also affected but not shown) demonstrates multiple superficial ulcers. Note the normal appearance to the transverse colon.

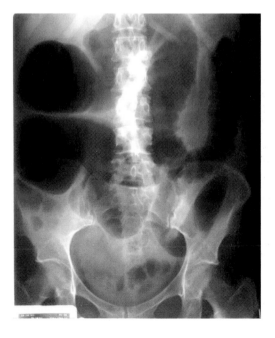

Fig. 2.28 Ulcerative colitis – megacolon. Fulminant colitis with dilatation of the transverse colon of more than 5.5 cm; at risk of perforation.

Table 2.1 Features of inflammatory bowel disease

Features	Crohn's disease	Ulcerative colitis
Distribution	Anywhere in gastrointestinal tract, mainly terminal ileum	Predominantly colon and rectum
Morphology	Skip lesions, aphthous ulcers, deep (rose thorn)	Disease involve continuous segments, superficial ulceration, aphthous ulcers (Fig. 2.27)
Fistula and sinuses	Common	Uncommon
Strictures	Yes	Relatively more common
Toxic dilatation	Uncommon	Common (Fig. 2.28)
Rectal involvement	Less than 50%	Greater than 95%
Anal fistula, sinus and fissures	Common	Uncommon
Terminal ileum	Narrowed, fissured	Dilated with a gaping ileo-caecal valve
Cancer risk	Uncommon	High
Pseudodiverticulation	Common	Not seen
Inflammatory polyps	Rare	Seen in about 20%
Gallstones	Common especially after surgery	No significant increase

Question 14

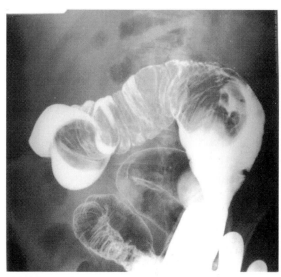

Age 66.
This patient presented with persistent vomiting and abdominal pain.

■ What are the radiological findings (Fig. 2.29)?

■ What is the diagnosis?

■ What further management would you suggest?

2

Fig. 2.29 Quiz case.

Answer

Barium has passed only as far as the proximal transverse colon, there is a large tubular filling defect within the transverse colon and a small polypoid lesion is present in the descending colon. The appearance are characteristic of a colo-colic intussusception. The radiological appearances of intussusception are said to resemble a coiled spring pattern.

At surgery, this lesion was found to be a caecal tumor at the lead point of the intussusception. A second 1.5 cm sigmoid colonic polyp was also present.

Colo-colic intussusception

Further management would include referral to a surgical team to consider urgent intervention. Staging of the tumour with CT will be required.

In adults, up to 80% of intussusceptions are secondary to a specific cause and approximately one-fifth are due to malignant neoplasms. Further causes include benign tumours, lipoma, Meckel's diverticulum and idiopathic.

Question 15

86-year-old female patient.
Unwell, pyrexia. Elevated white blood count.

■ What are the therapeutic options for this lesion (Fig. 2.30)?

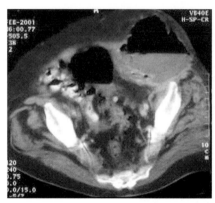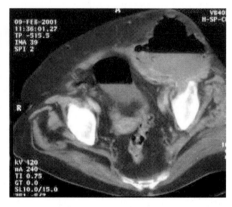

Fig. 2.30 Quiz case.

Answer

Diverticular abscess

There is a 10–12 cm abscess cavity with an air–fluid level in the left flank. Immediately adjacent to the abscess is a loop of bowel affected by diverticular disease with signs of direct communication.

Therapeutic options are either to insert a drainage tube under CT or ultrasound guidance or to proceed to laparotomy. If there is a large fistulous communication, then the surgical option would be favoured. Although the origin of the abscess is probably diverticular, the differential diagnosis includes a perforating colonic tumour and Crohn's colitis.

Colonic diverticulosis is an acquired herniation of the colonic mucosa and submucosa through the muscle layers. It is a condition more prevalent in developed countries with up to 50% of individuals affected by the seventh decade. The aetiology is linked to a diet lacking in roughage. The sigmoid is most frequently affected.

Complications include diverticular haemorrhage, colonic diverticulitis (Table 2.2), abscess formation, perforation, fistula and colonic stricture formation (see Fig. 2.31).

Table 2.2 **Colonic diverticulitis CT features**

- Diverticula often visible on CT as round oval focus protruding from bowel wall (may fill with oral contrast)
- Streaky peri-colic fat
- Bowel wall thickening
- Intestinal obstruction
- Fluid or gas in peritoneum
- Fistulation into
  - Bladder (look for an air–fluid level)
  - Small bowel/vagina/cutaneous
- Abscess or peri-colic collection

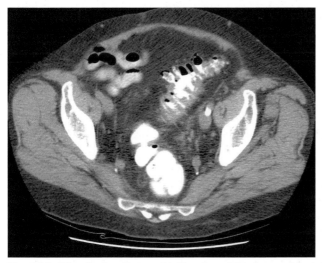

Fig. 2.31 Diverticular disease CT. The sigmoid colon wall is thickened and there are multiple diverticula. Note oral contrast in sigmoid colon.

Question 16

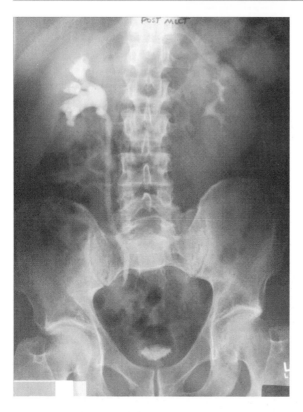

41-year-old male patient.
2-day history of right loin pain.

■ What does the film (Fig. 2.32) demonstrate?

■ What further film is required to make the diagnosis?

Fig. 2.32 Quiz case.

Answer

Obstructed right ureter

This film is the post-micturition film of an IVP series. It shows mild hydronephrosis of the right kidney and a mildly dilated right ureter. Contrast is seen as far as the right sacral region but no further. This indicates the level of obstruction of the ureter. The commonest cause of ureteric obstruction is stone disease. A preliminary/control film (prior to the administration of contrast) is necessary to check for the presence of radio-opaque calculus at the level of obstruction.

Causes of intraluminal ureteric obstruction

■ Opaque calculus (calcium stones).

■ Non-opaque calculus (uric acid, xanthine stones).

■ Blood clot.

■ Papillary necrosis.

■ Fungus ball.

Question 17

77-year-old female.
Progressive abdominal pain in left flank for 3 months.
Haematuria.

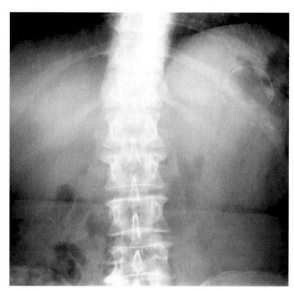

- Describe the appearances of the abdominal film (Fig. 2.33) and the CT scan (Figs 2.34 and 2.35).

- Where are the common sites for metastatic spread?

- What haematological problems can this cause?

2

Fig. 2.33 Quiz case.

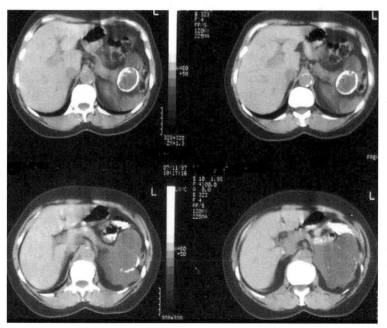

Fig. 2.34 Quiz case.

2

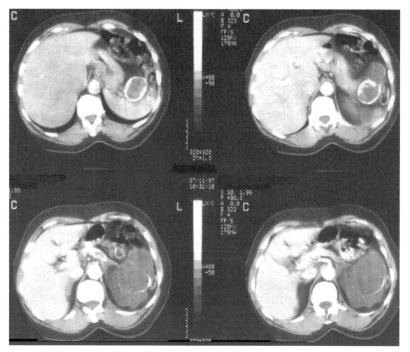

Fig. 2.35 Quiz case.

Answer

Renal cell carcinoma

On the plain film there is an area of curvilinear calcification in the left upper quadrant. From the CT scan it is clear that there is a large partly calcified renal mass of irregular outline. The appearances are of a calcified renal cell carcinoma. Staging requires an assessment of the local extent of tumour, local invasion to surrounding structures and assessment of the renal vein and IVC: tumour/thrombus extending into the renal vein and inferior vena cava are frequent features. Metastases occur to lung (pulmonary nodules), bone (lytic lesions) and regional lymph nodes.

Polycythaemia can result due to erythropoietin production by tumour. Hypercalcaemia is a recognised finding due to a PTH-like hormone (Table 2.3).

Table 2.3 Causes of renal calcification

Renal calculi
- Irregular calcification
  - TB
  - Carcinoma
  - Renal artery calcification

Nephrocalcinosis (renal parenchymal calcification)
- Medullary
  - Medullary sponge kidney
  - Renal tubular acidosis
  - Hypercalcaemia

- Cortical
  - Transplant failure
  - Acute cortical necrosis

Question 18

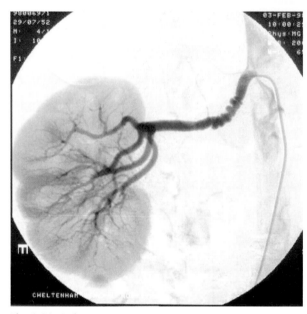

26-year-old female. Poorly controlled hypertension.

■ What is the diagnosis (Fig. 2.36)?

■ What is the radiological treatment?

■ What pharmacological agents should be avoided?

Fig. 2.36 Quiz case.

Answer

Renal artery stenosis

This selective renal artery arteriogram demonstrates the string of beads sign, which is characteristic of fibromuscular dysplasia of the renal artery. There are alternating areas of stenosis and aneurysm.

This is the commonest cause of renovascular hypertension in young adults and children. There is a female predominance. The renal arteries are not exclusively involved and the carotid vessels or other aortic branches are also affected, but less commonly than the renal arteries. The mid- and distal portions of the artery are affected whereas in atheromatous disease it is the proximal portion of the artery or the ostium which is involved.

Baloon angioplasty has a 90% success rate with a low restenosis rate (much less than with atheromatous disease).

ACE inhibitors are contraindicated in the treatment of hypertension in patients with renal artery stenosis. Non-steroidal anti-inflammatory drugs should be avoided.

Question 19

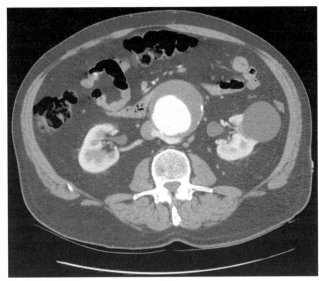

72-year-old male. Pulsatile mass in abdomen (Fig. 2.37).

■ What is the diagnosis?

■ What are the treatment options?

2

Fig. 2.37 Quiz case.

Answer

Abdominal aortic aneurysm

This is usually regarded as an aorta of greater than 3 cm diameter and is most prevalent in elderly men. The mortality of emergency surgical repair is 50% but only 5% if performed electively.

The risk of rupture increases as the size of the aneurysm expands. In the case of small aneurysms, regular ultrasound surveillance for every 6 months is recommended. The UK small aneurysms trial (4.0–5.5 cm aneurysms) showed no benefit in overall mortality for those offered early surgery. Indications for surgery include rupture, symptomatic aneurysms, rapid expansion and asymptomatic aneurysms over 6 cm (although the size is controversial).

Endovascular aneurysm repair prevents the need for laparotomy and aortic cross-clamping. A prosthetic graft is placed within the lumen via a femoral or iliac artery approach. Aorto-aortic, bifurcated aorto-iliac or aorto-uniiliac (with femero-femoral crossover) prostheses exist. Proximal and distal cuffs anchor the prosthesis in place and a tight seal aims to exclude the aneurysm from the circulation. Only 40% of aneurysms have a suitable morphology for this type of repair. If successfully excluded from the circulation, a reduction in aneurysm expansion is achieved.

Imaging of aneurysms should provide information on

- aneurysm size,

- proximal extent of the aneurysm to determine the site of clamping of the aorta (origin of the renal arteries),

- the course of the renal vein (retroaortic) (see Fig. 2.37),

- extension into iliac arteries.

Question 20

Male patient aged 53.
Alcoholic.
36 hours of severe abdominal pain.
Admitted to the intensive care unit following presentation to the accident and emergency unit where he had blood pressure 90/50, elevated amylase and hypocalcaemia.

■ What does the CT scan (Fig. 2.38) show?

■ How can the severity of this condition be graded?

■ What are the predisposing factors and the complications?

2

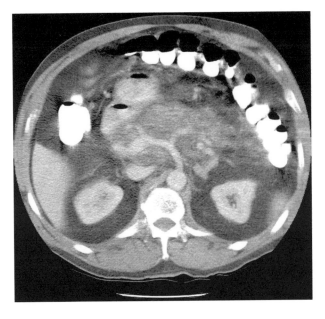

Fig. 2.38 Quiz case.

Answer

Acute pancreatitis

The pancreas is swollen and oedematous and has failed to enhance following intravenous contrast media. There is streaky increased density in the fat adjacent to the pancreatic tissues, the appearances are of diffuse acute pancreatitis.

Imaging

Ultrasound is frequently used to investigate patients with acute abdominal pain but overlying bowel gas often limits the ability to visualise the entire pancreatic gland. Its main use in the setting of acute pancreatitis is to evaluate the gall bladder and biliary tree to detect gallstones. It is also useful in the evaluation of pseudocyst or fluid collection.

2

CT has good specificity in diagnosing pancreatitis, although in up to one-third of patients with acute pancreatitis (especially mild pancreatitis) no detectable change in the size or appearance of the pancreas is evident. The CT appearances range from normal, gland enlargement, peripancreatic inflammation, single fluid collection and multiple fluid collections. Work has been done to try and predict (on the basis of CT) which patients are at greater risk of fatal pancreatitis. The key criteria is the presence of pancreatic necrosis. Pancreatic necrosis can be diagnosed when segments of the pancreas fail to enhance on contrast enhanced CT. The site of pancreatic necrosis can further predict disease severity. The presence of peripancreatic fluid collections is also associated with poor prognosis.

Severity assessment of acute pancreatitis

Early identification of patients with potentially severe acute pancreatitis is important as patients with delayed transfer to intensive care units have higher mortality.

Scoring systems

Several clinico-biochemical scoring systems exist for the assessment of the severity of acute pancreatitis. These are designed to predict the severity of clinical course in an individual patient, e.g. the Ransom criteria. The Ransom criteria comprise 11 criteria requiring up to 48 hours to be collected.

Ranson criteria[1]

Age greater than 55.
On admission

- Blood glucose >10 mmol/L

- WCC >16

- Lactate dehydrogenase >350 IU/L

- Aspartate transaminase >250 IU/L

Within 48 hours

- HCT decrease >10%

- Serum urea increase >0.7 mmol/L

- Serum Ca^{2+} <2 mmol/L

- Fluid sequestered >6 L

- PaO_2 <8 kPa

- Base deficit >4 mmol/L

Management

Supportive care is necessary with close clinical observation and early identification of complications. Patients with severe acute pancreatitis require early transfer to the intensive care unit and invasive monitoring. Treatment is mainly supportive and includes IV fluid and electrolyte replacement, nutritional support and analgesia, and support of respiratory dysfunction. Antibiotics and drugs aimed at reducing pancreatic secretions are of no proven value. Strategies such as peritoneal lavage, fresh frozen plasma, gabexate and H_2 blockers have been tried and their use is unproven. New treatments focusing on the cytokine cascade are currently under investigation. Indications for intervention include impacted gallstones, complicated pseudocyst, pancreatic abscess and infected necrosis.

Causes

- Gallstones: 30–40%
- Alcohol: 30–40%
- Hypercalcaemia: 10%
- Infections: CMV, mumps
- Congenital anatomical anomalies: pancreas divisum
- Trauma/post-ERCP
- Drugs: contraceptive pill, steroids
- Idiopathic: 10%
- Other metabolic causes: hyperlipidaemia type I and V
- Hereditary pancreatitis (affects children).

Systemic complications

- Hypotension
- Respiratory failure (15–55%): atelectasis, pneumonia, pleural effusions, ARDS
- Renal failure
- Metabolic: hypocalcaemia
- Coagulopathy: disseminated intravascular coagulation.

Local complications

- Pseudocyst formation 10% (Fig. 2.39).
- Abscess: in 10%, 2–4 weeks following severe pancreatitis – *E. coli*
- Fistula formation

121

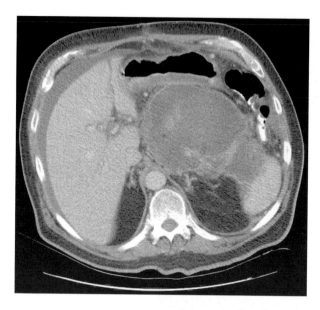

Fig. 2.39 Pseudocyst. Large fluid-filled pseudocyst anterior to pancreas.

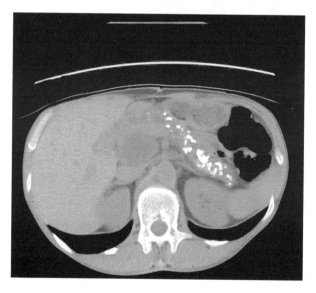

Fig. 2.40 Chronic pancreatitis and pseudocyst. Note the dense amorphous calcification throughout the pancreas.

- Biliary obstruction

- Haemorrhage

- Splenic artery pseudoaneurysm: in up to 10% of severe pancreatitis
  - Enzymatic errosion of splenic artery: may rupture into pseudocyst

- Splenic vein thrombosis.

Pseudocyst formation is not limited to acute pancreatitis and may follow chronic pancreatitis (see Fig. 2.40).

Question 21

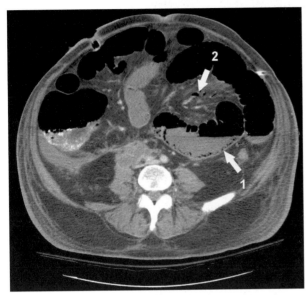

34-year-old male patient. Ventilated on intensive care. Septic and hypotensive. Blood pressure maintained with inotropes including noradrenaline.

■ What does the CT scan (Fig. 2.41) show?

Fig. 2.41 Quiz case.

Answer

Small bowel infarction

There are multiple tiny bubbles of gas in the wall of the small bowel – pneumatosis intestinalis (arrow 1). There is gas in the mesenteric veins (arrow 2) and the bowel is mildly dilated and filled with fluid. Portal vein gas is a further sign seen in up to one-third of patients. This is seen peripherally in the liver whereas pneumobilia is more central.

Predisposing factors include cardiovascular disease, acute hypotension, arrhythmia and thrombotic states. Noradrenaline can be associated with small bowel infarction as it may divert blood flow away from the bowel. Signs include abdominal pain, diarrhoea (often blood stained), persistent acidosis with an increasing base deficit despite fluid resuscitation, a rising lactate and an elevated white blood count with left shift.

The prognosis for small bowel infarction is grave with a very high mortality. Further radiological signs include bowel wall thickening and occasionally filling defects/thrombus can be identified in the superior mesenteric artery or vein.

References
1. J.H.C. Ranson *et al.* Prognostic signs and the role of operative management in acute Pancreatitis. Surgery, Gynecology and obstetrics 1974; 139: 69–81.

3

Trauma radiology

Chest trauma: case illustrations

Question 1

47-year-old male.
High speed road traffic accident.
Chest pain, breathless.
You are asked to assist in the emergency unit with a view to admission to intensive care. A chest drain has already been placed.
Widened mediastinum on the chest X-ray.
A CT scan of the chest (Figs 3.1 and 3.2) was performed.

■ What are the injuries?

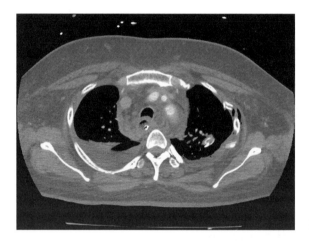

Fig. 3.1 Quiz case.

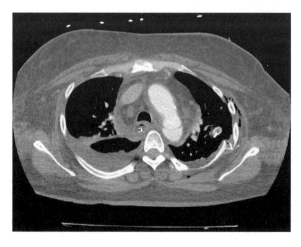

Fig. 3.2 Quiz case.

Answer

Traumatic aortic injury

Traumatic aortic injury is a major cause of mortality in patients with blunt thoracic trauma. The commonest cause is motor vehicle accidents, but also includes falls and blast injuries, the common mechanism being deceleration. About 80–90% of patients who sustain this injury die prior to hospital admission. Most patients who reach hospital alive have a tear at the aortic isthmus just distal to the subclavian artery. The injury is caused by shearing stress between the aortic arch, which is relatively fixed and the more mobile descending aorta.

Rapid diagnosis and surgical treatment is essential as 40% of patients will die within 24 hours without treatment.

Clinical signs include upper limb hypertension (due to acute coarctation effect) and wide pulse pressure. In patients, who survive aortic injury,

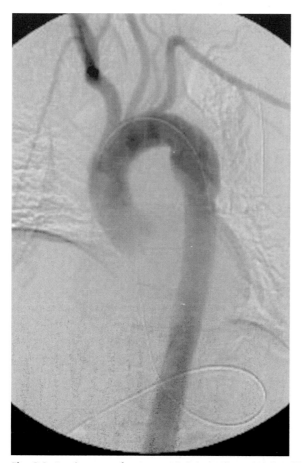

Fig. 3.3 Angiogram of acute aortic injury. There is a focal bulge immediately distal to left subclavian artery. This is a typical site for acute aortic injury seen in deceleration accidents.

the integrity of the aorta is often maintained only by the adventitia. Widening of the mediastinum on chest X-ray is caused by mediastinal blood. This is not usually due to aortic bleeding as this leads to sudden death. Mediastinal blood can come from injury to other vessels, e.g. azygous, paraspinal vessels. The great utility of the chest X-ray is not in diagnosing acute aortic injury but in excluding it. A normal chest X-ray has a negative predictive value of 98%. Numerous signs on the chest X-ray have been described in association with traumatic aortic injury. These signs are identified secondary to the associated mediastinal haematoma rather than the aortic injury itself. The signs include rightward tracheal shift, rightward deviation of any nasogastric tube, right paratracheal widening and widening of the paraspinal lines. Two of the most valuable signs are loss of contour of the aortic arch and contour abnormalities of the superior mediastinum, mediastinal widening, upper rib fractures, a left apical pleural cap are further recognised signs.

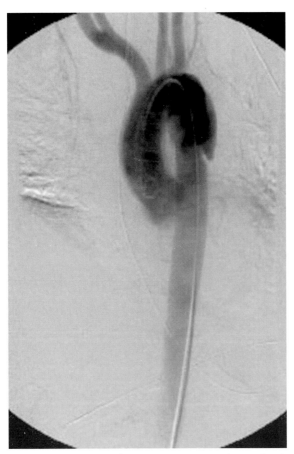

Fig. 3.4 Angiogram of acute aortic injury. This projection has been chosen to best illustrate the dissection/intimal flap which is seen projecting into the aortic lumen. This corresponds to the intimal flap seen on the contrast enhanced CT (Fig. 3.2).

Further investigation should be undertaken if aortic injury is suspected. There is debate regarding the place of contrast enhanced CT and angiography. CT is an excellent way of identifying mediastinal haematoma; it will visualise contour abnormalities of the aorta. The example above (Figs 3.1 and 3.2) demonstrates acute aortic injury with mediastinal blood and an intimal flap within the lumen of the aorta. In addition, there are rib fractures and pleural effusions.

Angiography has traditionally been regarded as the standard reference technique for evaluating patients with traumatic aortic injury. The typical appearance of acute aortic injury is demonstrated in Figs 3.3 and 3.4. There is abnormal outpouching of the aorta just distal to the origin of the left subclavian artery. The angiographic appearance is of a contained pseudoaneurysm. In addition, there is a linear component due to an intimal flap seen distal to the pseudoaneurysm.

Treatment is with prompt surgical repair. Control of blood pressure is advised until surgical repair can be accomplished.

3

Question 2

A call has come from a paramedic team that a male aged 38 is shortly arriving in the emergency unit. He has sustained steering wheel injuries to the chest following a high speed motor vehicle accident.

- How are you going to deal with the initial assessment and management?
- What does the CT scan (Fig. 3.5) show?
- What are the main injuries sustained in blunt chest trauma?

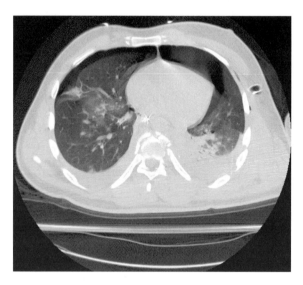

Fig. 3.5 Quiz case.

Answer

Initial assessment and management should follow Advanced Trauma Life Support (ATLS) guidelines [1] – A, B, C, D, E. A cervical spine injury should be assumed in any patient with multi-system trauma.

Airway maintenance (with cervical spine control)

Speak to the patient – do they respond? If the patient is able to communicate verbally the airway is unlikely to be in immediate danger. Repeated assessment of airway patency should still be performed. All patients must receive oxygen (10–15 L/min from a reservoir bag if breathing spontaneously). If airway obstruction is present simple measures to clear the airway, chin lift or jaw thrust, should be undertaken immediately. Reduced conscious level (Glasgow Coma Score of 8 or less) airway disruption or inability to oxygenate the patient by face mask indicate the need for a definitive airway. Endotracheal intubation (with stabilisation of the cervical spine) can be performed with a rapid sequence induction and cricoid pressure, or with awake fibre-optic intubation depending on the clinical circumstances. When assessing and managing the airway in patient's with blunt chest trauma it is important to look for other injuries to the head, face, cervical spine, and potential sites of injury to the larynx, trachea or lower airway. Laryngeal or tracheal injury may require placement of a surgical airway below the level of the injury.

Breathing and ventilation

A careful physical examination of ventilatory function is particularly important in chest injured patients. This should include *inspection* of ventilatory rate and chest movement looking for paradoxical respiration and other obvious injuries. *Palpation* is important to identify crepitus from rib fractures, surgical emphysema and areas of focal tenderness. *Auscultation* should be performed with particular reference to signs of pneumo- or haemothorax. *Percussion* may demonstrate the presence of blood or air in the chest.

Assess, oxygenate and ventilate as necessary. Injuries that acutely impair ventilation are tension pneumothorax, flail chest with pulmonary contusion, massive haemothorax and open pneumothorax. These should be treated as found, a tension pneumothorax is a life-threatening emergency which must be treated immediately, X-ray confirmation should *not* be sought.

Circulation

The main causes of hypotension in the setting of blunt thoracic trauma are hypovolaemia, pneumothorax, cardiac tamponade and myocardial contusion. Haemorrhage is the predominant cause of post-injury deaths that are preventable. Hypotension following injury must be considered to be hypovolaemic in origin until otherwise proven. Fluid should be given (2 L of warmed Hartmann's solution) through large peripheral cannula while the underlying aetiologies are explored. The presence of cardiac arrhythmias should raise the possibility of cardiac contusion. A central line may be needed for therapy and monitoring.

Disability (neurologic evaluation)

A rapid neurological examination can be based on

- *A* alert,

- *V* respond to vocal stimuli,

- *P* respond only to painful stimuli,

- *U* unresponsive to stimuli and assessment of the patient's pupils.

Exposure/environmental control

The patient should then be completely undressed for thorough examination and assessment. Attention must be paid to maintenance of the patient's temperature.

Aggressive resuscitation and the management of life-threatening injuries, as they are identified, are essential to maximise patient survival.

X-rays should be used judiciously and should *not* delay patient resuscitation. The AP chest film and AP pelvis may provide information that can guide resuscitation of the patient with blunt trauma. Chest X-rays may detect potentially life-threatening injuries that require treatment and pelvic films may demonstrate fractures of the pelvis that indicate the need for early blood transfusion. A lateral cervical spine X-ray that demonstrates an injury is an important finding, whereas a negative or inadequate film does not exclude cervical spine injury. These films can be taken in the resuscitation area, usually with a portable X-ray unit, but should not interrupt the resuscitation process.

Blunt chest trauma (see Fig. 3.5)
The example demonstrates bilateral pleural effusions, a left pneumothorax, contusion of the left lung and a left-sided chest tube. There is also a burst fracture of T9 vertebral body. This is seen in sagittal section in Fig. 3.6. Blunt thoracic trauma such as steering wheel injury has a high potential for causing life-threatening thoracic injuries. Approximately 20% of trauma-related deaths are attributable to chest injuries. The mechanisms include rapid deceleration, direct impact and compression. Systematic evaluation of the chest X-ray is an important facet of early management after the primary survey and initial resuscitation.

The chest X-ray or CT for blunt trauma can be divided into systems for the purposes of ensuring that all areas are looked at.

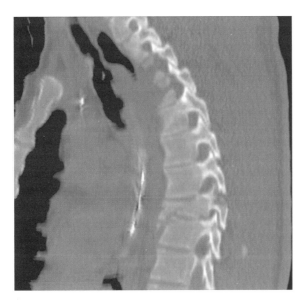

Fig. 3.6 Chest trauma. Thoracic spine reconstruction sagital plane. This shows a burst fracture also seen on axial images (see Fig. 3.5).

Potential sites of injury in blunt chest trauma

Skeleton

Rib fractures   The positive identification of rib fractures means that the underlying lung must be examined for contusions, haemothorax, pneumothorax or laceration (Figs 3.7 and 3.8). The presence of multiple fractures or the combination of anterior and posterior fractures can cause a flail segment (see Fig. 3.9). The upper ribs (1–3) are protected by the bony

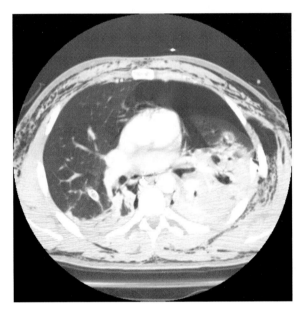

3

Fig. 3.7 Chest trauma. There is extensive contusion involving the left lung, a left-sided pneumothorax and extensive subcutaneous emphysema. Several pockets of gas are noted within the left lung contusion at the level of a left-sided rib fracture; these are pulmonary lacerations.

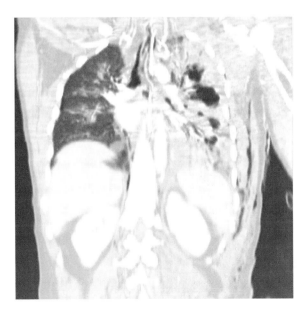

Fig. 3.8 Chest trauma. CT coronal reformat. Pulmonary contusion and laceration. There is extensive opacification of the left hemithorax with several air-filled pockets indicating the site of pulmonary laceration.

133

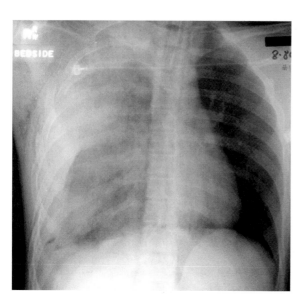

Fig. 3.9 Flail chest. The diagnosis is made by observing paradoxical chest wall movement in combination with multiple right-sided rib fractures on the chest X-ray. Note the surgical emphysema and lung contusion.

framework of the upper limb. The scapula, humerus, and clavicle, along with their muscular attachments provide a barrier to rib injury. Fractures of the scapula, first or second ribs, or the sternum suggest a magnitude of injury that place the head, neck, spinal cord, lungs and great vessels at risk for serious associated injury. Because of the severity of the associated injuries, mortality can be as high as 35%. Pain from rib fractures can precipitate hypoventilation and atelectasis. Adequate analgesia is essential.

Flail chest (Fig. 3.9)

In a flail chest injury paradoxical motion of the free-floating segment of chest wall occurs during respiration. This means that during inspiration the affected segment moves inwards in the opposite direction to the rest of the thoracic cage. Lateral chest wall injuries are the commonest cause and the injury usually consists of fractures in at least two sites in multiple adjacent ribs. If the pulmonary condition worsens, the paradoxical movement of the chest wall becomes more severe, making respiration more inefficient. In the unconscious patient the chest wall muscles do not splint the area and the flail effect is more pronounced.

The diagnosis is clinical and depends upon recognising paradoxical chest wall movement in the presence of multiple fractures on the chest X-ray. Ventilation is impaired, coughing is ineffective and the injuries are usually very painful. This injury should not be underestimated, assisted ventilation may be necessary. The patient should be monitored and observed in an HDU or ITU. Thoracic epidural analgesia is often used to provide pain relief to facilitate respiration and clearing of secretions.

Thoracic spine

Make a point of tracing the contour of the thoracic spine on the frontal radiograph. Reconstructions can be performed from spiral CT (see Fig. 3.6).

The most common fractures are anterior compression fractures and burst fractures, most of which occur at the thoraco-lumbar junction.

Check for shoulder dislocation, clavicle or scapulae fractures and sternal injuries.

Pulmonary contusion

Pulmonary contusion is defined as focal injury with oedema, alveolar and interstitial haemorrhage. It is the most common potentially lethal chest injury. The respiratory failure may be subtle and develops over time rather than occurring instantaneously. Patients need careful monitoring and re-evaluation for several days after the injury.

The initial presentation is usually with hypoxia and on the X-ray or CT, the pattern is of air space shadowing (Fig. 3.9). This is normally non-segmental, often peripheral and adjacent to the area of trauma. Other causes of air space shadowing seen in trauma patients include aspiration, atelectasis and pulmonary oedema (cardiogenic and non-cardiogenic). Management is with oxygen therapy either with a positive pressure mask or mechanical ventilation. Due to the high force required to cause contusion there are often other accompanying injuries. In contrast, due to the increased compliance of the chest in children, pulmonary contusion can occur in the absence of rib fractures.

Pulmonary laceration can occur secondary to shear forces in blunt trauma (Figs 3.7 and 3.8) or in penetrating injury. This is easy to miss if there is surrounding contusion. It is characterised by collections of air within surrounding contusion.

Pneumothorax

There must be a high index of suspicion for pneumothorax in blunt chest trauma – it occurs in over one-third of cases. If there are clinical suspicions of tension (tracheal deviation, dilated neck veins, hyper-resonant percussion note over one hemithorax and absent breath sounds, hypoxia and hypotension) then the chest must be decompressed immediately by inserting a large bore needle into the second intercostal space in the mid-clavicular line of the affected hemithorax. This must be done before obtaining a chest X-ray. Subsequent chest drain insertion is usually performed in the fourth or fifth interspace in the mid-axillary line. Even small pneumothoraces can be clinically relevant in the setting of trauma, as ventilation or general anaesthesia may become necessary.

Haemothorax

Large volumes of blood can accumulate in the pleural space and this can cause hypovolaemia as well as ventilatory problems from the mass effect. Sites of bleeding include intercostal vessels, internal mammary artery the mediastinal great vessels or abdominal viscera in the presence of diaphragmatic rupture. The diagnosis is made by identifying fluid on the X-ray and sampling the fluid in the pleural space.

Massive haemothorax results from a rapid accumulation of more than 1500 ml of blood in the chest cavity. It is most commonly caused by a penetrating wound that dirupts the systemic or hilar vessels. It may also result from blunt trauma.

Cardiac injury

The most anterior of the heart chambers – the right ventricle and right atrium are the most frequently injured. A combination of cardiac enzyme elevation, ECG changes (usually significant conduction abnormalities), echocardiography and thallium scintigraphy can be used to assess cardiac contusion.

Pericardial tamponade

This is seen more often in association with penetrating trauma. Clinical signs are unreliable in the resuscitation setting but can include venous pressure elevation, hypotension and muffled heart sounds. Prompt transthoracic echocardiography may be a valuable way of assessing the pericardium but has a false negative rate of about 5%. Examination of the pericardial sac may form part of a focused abdominal ultrasound examination performed by a trauma team properly trained in its use. If found, pericardial tamponade frequently requires drainage. Underlying causes include cardiac rupture, aortic disruption and cardiac contusion.

Blunt abdominal and pelvic trauma: case illustrations

Question 3

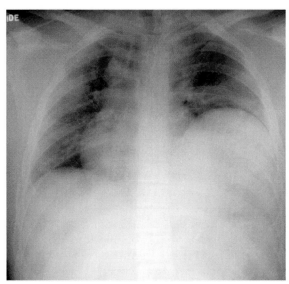

Fig. 3.10 Quiz case.

53-year-old male patient.
Assessed in the emergency department following motor vehicle accident.
Splenic laceration diagnosed on ultrasound scan.
Progressive deterioration in respiratory function.

3

■ What do the X-rays (Figs 3.10 and 3.11) which were taken 8 hours apart demonstrate?

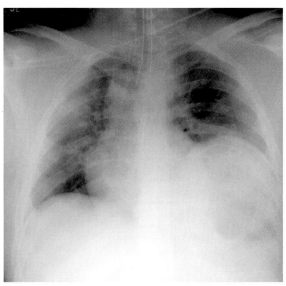

Fig. 3.11 Quiz case.

Answer

Diaphragmatic rupture

There is an opacity in the left hemithorax above the left hemidiaphragm on the first film. The second film demonstrates a nasogastric tube above the diaphragm in the stomach [verified after CT (Fig. 3.12)]. This has passed into the left hemithorax through a rupture in the left hemidiaphragm.

Diaphragmatic rupture can follow either blunt or penetrating abdominal trauma but patients may be asymptomatic for months or years

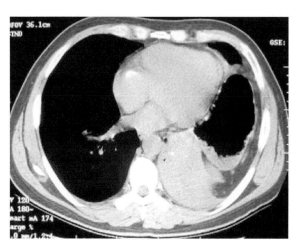

Fig. 3.12 Diaphragm rupture CT. The stomach and mesenteric fat has herniated into the left hemithorax. Other signs of traumatic diaphragmatic rupture on CT include discontinuity of hemidiaphragm/abnormal contour, herniation of colon, small bowel or abdominal contents into chest.

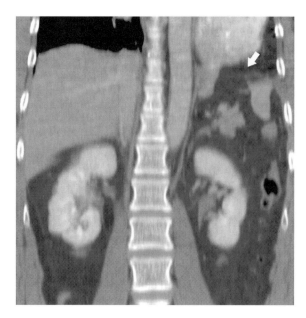

Fig. 3.13 Diaphragm rupture. Coronal reformat. The outline of the diaphragm is lost and the stomach is seen herniated into the left hemithorax.

following trauma. Up to 90% of diaphragmatic ruptures diagnosed are left sided. Injuries frequently associated with diaphragmatic rupture include

■ fracture of lower ribs,

■ perforation of hollow viscus,

■ rupture of spleen.

Diaphragm rupture can be a difficult diagnosis to make. When gross, chest X-ray changes include bowel loops, nasogastric tube present in the chest, but signs may only be subtle such as loss of contour of the diaphragm silhouette. If there is herniation of a hollow viscus into the chest there may be constriction at the point of herniation – collar sign. The most common finding on CT is abrupt discontinuity of the diaphragm. Sagittal and coronal reformatted images can improve the sensitivity and specificity of CT in making the diagnosis (see Fig. 3.13).

3

Question 4

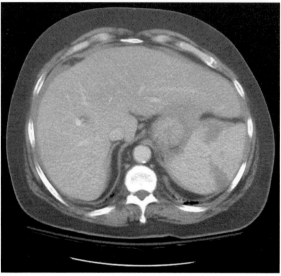

36-year-old male.
Road traffic accident.
Left upper quadrant
pain, free fluid seen on
ultrasound (Fig. 3.14).

■ What is the
management of this
condition?

Fig. 3.14 Quiz case.

Answer

Splenic laceration
The contrast enhanced CT scan shows a large splenic laceration with
haematoma in the left upper quadrant which is surrounding the spleen.

Management of blunt splenic trauma
The spleen is the most commonly injured organ in the abdomen.
Ultrasound can demonstrate splenic laceration, adjacent fluid (Fig. 3.15) or
splenic haematoma, but the technique is often limited by pain and patient
immobility. Contrast enhanced CT gives excellent visualisation of the left
upper quadrant and in many hospitals it is now the preferred modality of
imaging. It will also demonstrate any associated injuries, e.g. renal injury or
rib fractures. Just under a half of patients with splenic injury have
left-sided rib fractures. Splenic injury can be acute or delayed (usually due to
rupture of subcapsular haematoma). Delayed rupture is usually in the first
7–10 days following the injury. Injuries may occur inadvertently during
abdominal surgery or following trivial trauma especially if the spleen
is abnormal, e.g. malaria or infectious mononucleosis.

Surgical opinion varies regarding the need for splenectomy. Although
splenic trauma grading systems exist (Table 3.1) these are not a good
predictor of which patients require splenectomy.

The subsequent risk of pneumococcal infection means that surgical
splenectomy is avoided where possible. Patients with cardiovascular

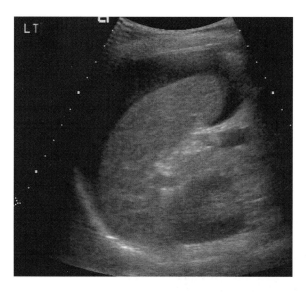

Fig. 3.15 Abdominal ultrasound demonstrating free peritoneal fluid. In the setting of blunt abdominal trauma this is usually haemoperitoneum.

Table 3.1 **Grading of splenic injury**

1. Minor subcapsular tear or haematoma

2. Parenchymal injury not extending to hilum

3. Injury involving vessels and hilum

4. Shattered spleen

instability require resuscitation and early surgery. Surgical options include splenectomy or splenic repair (splenic conservation needs to preserve more than 20% of tissue).

Approximately one-third of patients fail conservative management. Monitoring should include cardiovascular signs and haematocrit. Children can often be managed conservatively as they have an increased proportion of low grade injuries and they have fewer multiple injuries.

If conservative management is successful, then patients should have limited physical activity for 6 weeks and play no contact sports for 6 months. Complications following splenic trauma include recurrent bleeding, delayed rupture and pseudoaneurysm formation (Fig. 3.16). Pseudoaneurysm formation is a common cause for failure of non-operative management. This is diagnosed by identifying an intra-parenchymal contrast blush on CT or using angiography. Acute bleeding at the time of injury and delayed pseudoaneurysm formation can both be treated with coil embolisation (Fig. 3.17).

3

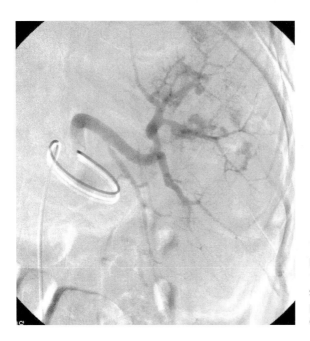

Fig. 3.16 Angiogram: 1 week following blunt splenic trauma. Multiple pseudoaneurysms are demonstrated.

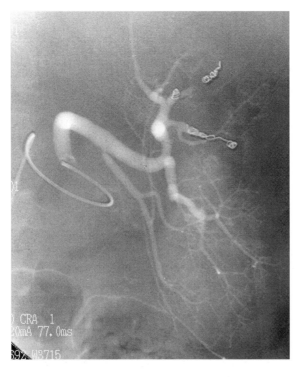

Fig. 3.17 Angiogram following coil embolisation of pseudoaneurysms. The spleen is preserved following blunt splenic trauma whenever possible to reduce the risk of subsequent infection. Aggressive imaging follow-up and coil embolisation have helped to reduce the rate of splenectomy for blunt abdominal trauma.

Question 5

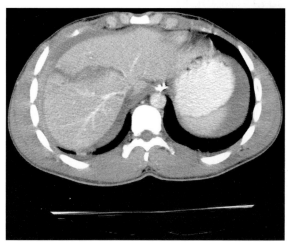

Male patient, age 41. Motor vehicle accident not wearing seat belt. Abdominal pain. On physical examination, the patient is shocked and there is abdominal guarding.

■ What does the CT (Fig. 3.18) show?

Fig. 3.18 Quiz case.

Answer

Liver trauma

The CT demonstrates an extensive liver laceration through the right lobe of the liver. There is widespread free fluid within the peritoneal space seen around the liver and also the spleen.

The liver is the second most commonly injured intra-abdominal organ. This is partly related to its large size, fixed position and relative friability. If the liver capsule is torn, intra-peritoneal haemorrhage can be extensive due to the rich dual blood supply of the liver. Delayed rupture is not encountered following liver trauma unlike splenic trauma. The most commonly injured site is the posterior segment of the right lobe. Left lobe injuries are less common but are associated with injuries of other retroperitoneal structures, e.g. duodenum and pancreas. On CT, liver lacerations appear as non-enhancing irregular, linear, round, or branching regions of low attenuation. Lacerations can extend to the visceral surface sometimes as irregular jagged lines. Intra-parenchymal haematomas appear as mass like, low density non-enhancing regions (Fig. 3.19). Subcapsular haematomas extend around the capsule in a lenticular pattern compressing the underlying liver. Periportal low density is frequently encountered in the setting of blunt abdominal trauma and has been linked to aggressive fluid resuscitation.

Surgical series have demonstrated that 80% of traumatic liver injuries can be treated conservatively unless there is haemodynamic instability. Active haemorrhage detected on CT can be treated by catheter embolisation. Complications following liver trauma include recurrent bleeding, pseudoaneurysm formation, bile duct injury, biloma and

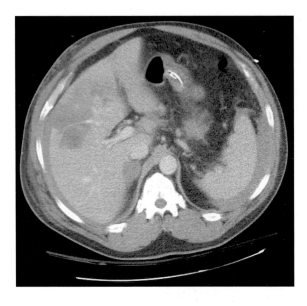

Fig. 3.19 Liver trauma. There is a large non-enhancing laceration/haematoma in the right lobe of liver with haemoperitoneum around both the liver and spleen.

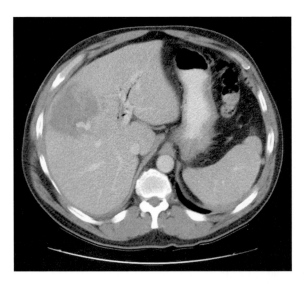

Fig. 3.20 Liver trauma, pseudoaneurysm. Dense intra-parenchymal contrast blush (in the arterial phase) adjacent to the liver haematoma – 8 days following the initial injury.

fistula formation, e.g. arterio-portal fistula. Pseudoaneurysms appear as intense foci of contrast enhancement seen best on arterial phase imaging (see Fig. 3.20). These can be treated with coil embolisation (see Figs 3.21 and 3.22). Early intervention with coil embolisation, percutaneous drainage, ERCP and stenting of bile duct injuries has helped reduce the proportion of patients requiring surgery following liver trauma.

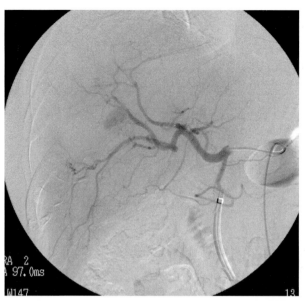

Fig. 3.21 Blunt abdominal trauma, liver trauma. Right hepatic artery angiogram demonstrating pseudoaneurysm.

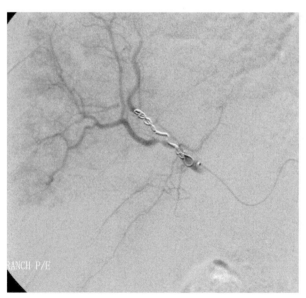

Fig. 3.22 Blunt abdominal trauma, liver trauma. Right hepatic artery angiogram following coil embolisation: demonstrating no filling of the previously identified pseudoaneurysm.

Question 6

28-year-old female patient.
Involved in high speed motor vehicle accident restrained by 'lap-type' seat belt.
On physical examination there is bruising in a lap belt distribution.

■ What does the imaging (Figs 3.23–3.25) show?

■ What other injuries should be considered?

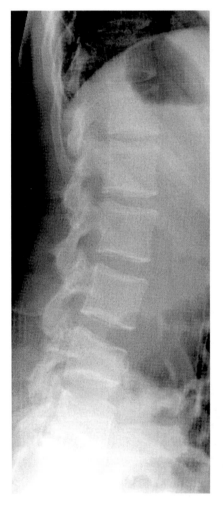

Fig. 3.23 Quiz case.

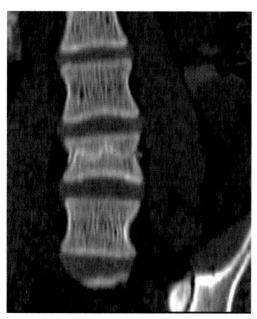

Fig. 3.24 Quiz case.

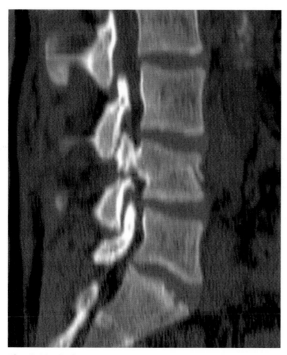

Fig. 3.25 Quiz case.

Answer

Chance fracture of L4

A chance fracture is commonly associated with use of 'lap-type' seat belts in high speed motor crashes. A chance fracture is a horizontal vertebral fracture caused by a flexion injury. The body bends around the fulcrum of the belt and causes an injury in the horizontal plane. The fracture line extends through the neural arch and vertebral body. A lateral X-ray or sagittal reconstruction best demonstrates the injury. Since the fracture runs in the axial plane, a routine axial CT may miss a chance fracture.

There is a high incidence of intra-abdominal injuries associated with chance fracture. Both solid organ (pancreas) and bowel injuries (duodenum) are associated with chance fracture. The abdominal CT scan of the same patient demonstrates jejunal small bowel thickening and extravasation of oral contrast medium in keeping with jejunal injury and perforation (see Fig. 3.26).

Clinical signs of bowel trauma may be absent, minimal or delayed beyond the first 24 hours. The small bowel contents are of neutral pH and sterile so do not induce rapid peritoneal signs. Morbidity and mortality from bowel injury increases if surgical intervention is delayed – this is especially true of duodenal injury. The CT findings of duodenal injury may be subtle with only tiny extraluminal gas bubbles, or minimal duodenal fold thickening. Small bowel injury usually occurs at points of fixation such as the ligament of Treitz or the ileo-caecal valve. Only the most minor small bowel or mesenteric injury can be treated with non-operative management. Signs on CT include wall thickening (due to haematoma), intra-peritoneal air, extravasation of oral contrast and sentinel clot adjacent to bowel. Intra-peritoneal air can be present in the absence of hollow viscus injury due to pneumothorax (via the diaphragm) or subcutaneous dissection from the chest.

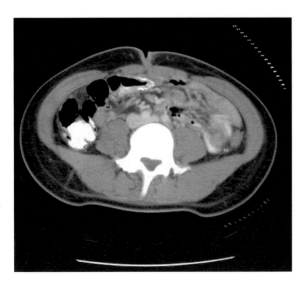

Fig. 3.26 Lap-type seat-belt injury: jejunal and mesenteric injury. In the left flank there is free contrast in the peritoneal space surrounding loops of small bowel. Solid organ or bowel injury should be 'expected' in the presence of a chance fracture.

Question 7

12-year-old girl.
Fall from horse. Pain in right upper quadrant.

- What is the diagnosis (Fig. 3.27)?

- How would you manage the case?

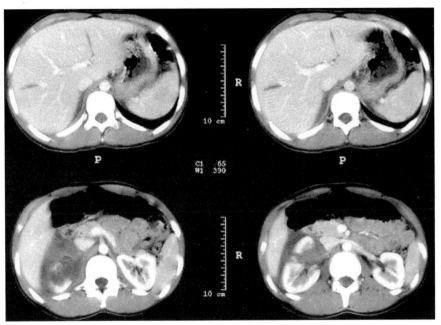

Fig. 3.27 Quiz case.

Answer

Blunt renal trauma
There is a laceration from the cortical surface through the parenchyma of the right kidney communicating with the hilum – renal fracture. There is perinephric haemorrhage and fluid surrounding the kidney. The kidney remains well perfused. In addition, there is a laceration through the right lobe of the liver.

The majority of renal injuries are from blunt trauma. Flank pain, bruising and haematuria can accompany renal trauma but are a poor indicator of the extent of disease. Renal pedicle injury or traumatic renal vein thrombosis can present with no associated haematuria. It is necessary to correlate clinical findings with the mechanism and severity of trauma.

The role of imaging is to assess the extent of injury – trauma grading (see Table 3.2) and to determine the function of the contralateral kidney.

Table 3.2 Grading of blunt renal trauma (American Association of Surgeons in Trauma)

1. Renal contusions and subcapsular haematoma

2. Cortical laceration less than 1 cm in depth and non-expanding perirenal haematomas

3. Parenchymal lesion extending more than 1 cm into renal substance, extension into the collecting system or evidence of urinary extravasation

4. Lacreation involving the collecting system, traumatic thrombosis of a segmental renal arterial branch, and injuries to the main renal artery not associated with renal devascularisation

5. Renal fragmentation or renovascular pedicle injury

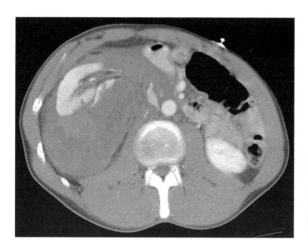

Fig. 3.28 Renal trauma. There is a large right-sided perinephric haematoma surrounding the right kidney which is displacing it anteriorly.

Contrast enhanced CT is the gold standard for assessing renal trauma (Fig. 3.28). Delayed CT images are important when imaging for renal trauma to check for urine leak. Renal lacerations are irregular low-density areas in the parenchyma.

Lacerations through the hilum which contact two cortical surfaces are termed fractures. The majority of renal injuries can be managed without the need for surgery even in the presence of major laceration or urine leak. Grades 1 and 2 are managed non-operatively with excellent results; patients have normal functioning kidneys on follow-up imaging. Most patients with grade 3 and 4 injuries are managed non-operatively. Close monitoring of patients with grade 3 and 4 injuries with use of percutaneous drainage and angiographic embolisation (Fig. 3.29) has reduced the laparotomy rate in this group. Moderate urine leaks can be managed conservatively with ureteric stenting. Persistent large

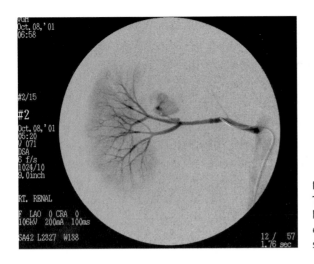

Fig. 3.29 Renal angiogram. There is active bleeding/contrast extravasation from a segmental renal artery.

urine leak, pelvi-ureteric junction avulsion, enlarging central or subcapsular haematoma, extensive avascularised parenchyma and shock in the presence of intra-peritoneal or retro-peritoneal haematoma need surgical intervention. Attempted salvage of a devascularised kidney is contraversial but may not be attempted if the contralateral kidney is normal.

Question 8

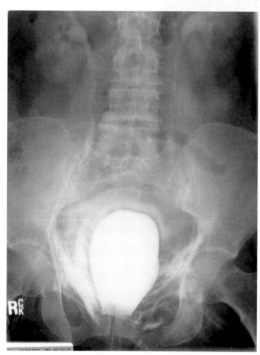

Male aged 28.
Road traffic accident.
Pelvic fractures on plain
radiograph (Fig. 3.30).
Frank haematuria.

- What is this study and
  what does it
  demonstrate?

Fig. 3.30 Quiz case.

Answer

Cystogram with extra-peritoneal bladder rupture. The cystogram
demonstrates extravasation of contrast into the extra-peritoneal space
around the bladder. Note the multiple pelvic fractures.

Lower genitourinary trauma

Bladder injuries are most common following blunt trauma and 85% are
associated with pelvic fractures. Urethral injury (particularly of the proximal
segment) is also usually associated with pelvic fracture and is mainly
a male problem. Pelvic pain, inability to void, high riding prostate on
PR examination, and haematuria are all clues to urethral or bladder trauma.

Bladder injuries are best classified as either intra-peritoneal (15–35%) or
extra-peritoneal (65–85%). Intra-peritoneal rupture is usually caused by a
burst injury of the bladder dome in a distended bladder and infrequently
by pelvic fractures. Extra-peritoneal injuries are associated with penetration
injury from pelvic fractures especially pubic bone fractures (95%).

Imaging investigations should include plain films to diagnose the
presence of pelvic fractures and a retrograde urethrogram if urethral injury
is suspected. The latter should be performed prior to Foley catheter
insertion (if urethral injury is suspected). A retrograde cystogram is a
reliable method of assessing the presence of bladder injury.

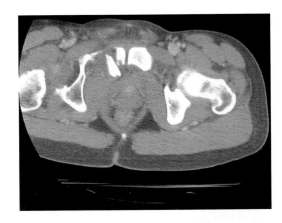

Fig. 3.31 Bladder trauma. Pelvic fractures should raise the suspicion of bladder trauma. Either delayed CT images or a CT cystogram can be performed.

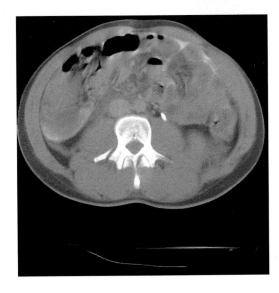

Fig. 3.32 Intra-peritoneal bladder rupture. Delayed CT imaging demonstrates dense contrast (excreted in the urine) in the peritoneal space. The normal mechanism is a blunt injury to the full bladder which ruptures into the peritoneal space.

Two hundred and fifty millilitres of water soluble contrast medium is introduced into the bladder through a Foley catheter and a further 150 ml if the patient does not experience any discomfort. CT cystography is often the most convenient method, as acute trauma patients often have additional indications for CT. Alternatively, fluoroscopy can be used when frontal and lateral views are obtained with images also taken post-void.

Flame-shaped extravasation superior and lateral to the bladder indicate extra-peritoneal rupture (see Fig. 3.30). Intra-peritoneal injury is manifested by contrast throughout the peritoneal cavity, outlining bowel and in the paracolic gutters. Delayed CT imaging may demonstrate bladder rupture and also any associated bony pelvic injuries (see Figs 3.31 and 3.32). It is less sensitive than cystography. The importance of identifying intra-peritoneal rupture is that surgical repair is required acutely. Extra-peritoneal ruptures are treated conservatively with catheter drainage and antibiotics unless a cystogram at 7–10 days demonstrates persistent leakage.

153

Question 9

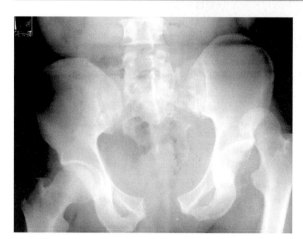

Male aged 29.
Road traffic accident.

■ What type of fracture is demonstrated (Fig. 3.33)?

■ What are the main complications from pelvic fractures?

Fig. 3.33 Quiz case.

Answer

Open book pelvic fracture with diastasis of the symphasis pubis and sacro-iliac joint. Dislocation of the left femur.

Considerable force is required to cause a pelvic fracture and there is a high association with injury to distant organs – brain injury, liver laceration, aortic disruption.

Complications of pelvic fractures

■ Haemorrhage: can be life threatening.

■ Bladder injury: consider cystogram.

■ Urethral injury: consider urethrogram (prior to bladder catheter insertion).

■ Prostate injury.

■ Vaginal injury.

■ Rectal and perineal injury.

■ Neurological injury.

■ Sepsis from bowel or urinary tract injury.

The pelvis is supplied by an extensive venous plexus and several major arteries. Initial managagement of a major pelvic disruption associated with haemorrhage requires haemorrhage control and rapid fluid resuscitation. Simple techniques such as wrapping the 'open book' pelvic injury in a sheet to try to stabilise the pelvic ring can temporarily improve

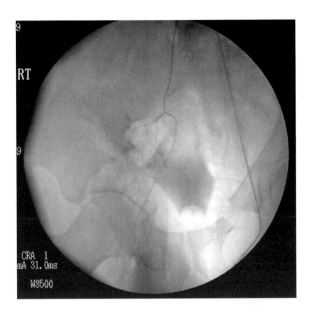

Fig. 3.34 Angiogram in patient with pelvic fracture demonstrating active bleeding. This was subsequently coiled.

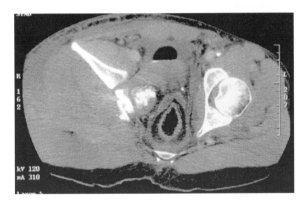

Fig. 3.35 Contrast enhanced CT scan. Note the right-sided pelvic fractures and the contrast extravasation from active bleeding.

haemostasis but control of haemodynamically unstable patients needs urgent surgery or angiography (Fig. 3.34). Pelvic surgery may decompress tamponaded retro-peritoneal haematoma and for this reason angiography may be preferred. Certain anatomical locations predispose to vessel injury (Fig. 3.35). Injuries of the sciatic notch, crush injuries of the sacrum and vertical shear injuries can all result in arterial tears.

Question 10

24-year-old man.
Motorcycle accident.

■ What complication (Figs 3.36 and 3.37) has occurred?

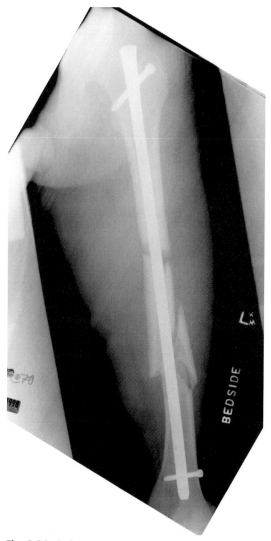

Fig. 3.36 Quiz case.

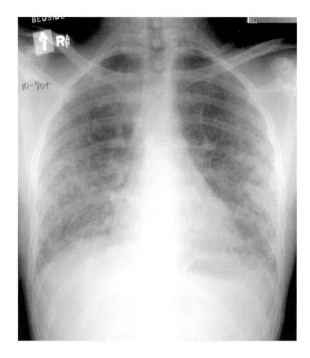

Fig. 3.37 Quiz case.

Answer

Femoral diaphysis fracture with fat embolism
As with pelvic fractures a significant force is required to fracture the femoral diaphysis – it is the strongest bone in the body. The femoral shaft has a rich blood supply and femoral fractures are often associated with considerable blood loss and haematoma formation.

Fat embolism
Fat embolism is usually associated with long bone or pelvic trauma, but can rarely be associated with parenteral lipid infusion or corticosteroid treatment. The traditional explanation is that fat droplets from the bone marrow escape into the venous system and pass to the lung (and the brain via arteriovenous shunts). A second explanation is that altered internal homeostasis in the severely traumatised patient causes systemic release of fatty acids and chylomicrons which subsequently coalesce to give fat embolisation. Fat embolisation is a clinical diagnosis. Clinical features include hypoxia, tachycardia and fever. Red/brown petechial spots may appear over the trunk and axillae and if present are virtually diagnostic. Retinal, subconjunctival and oral haemorrhages are also sometimes seen.

The chest X-ray shows bilateral diffuse pulmonary infiltrates which appear 24–48 hours following the clinical picture. The CT head appearance may be normal but can show white matter petechial haemorrhages or changes consistent with microvascular injury.

Treatment is supportive.

157

Complications of femoral fractures

- Haemorrhagic shock

- Vascular injury

- Neurological injury

- Infection (with open fractures)

- Respiratory complications
  - Fat embolism (see Fig. 3.37)
  - Adult respiratory distress syndrome

- DVT and pulmonary embolism

- Compartment syndrome (Fig. 3.38)

- Complications related to the fracture: shortening, malrotation, non/delayed union.

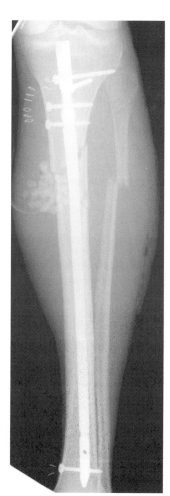

Fig. 3.38 Tibial fracture – compartment syndrome. Note the antibiotic beads and considerable soft tissue swelling. The patient later had a fasciotomy.

Compartment syndrome

Compartment syndrome (or Volkmann contracture) occurs when perfusion pressure falls below tissue pressure in a fixed volume body compartment. The condition is most frequently associated with long bone fracture (Fig. 3.38) particularly of the tibia but has also been described in several other body compartments including femur, upper limb, abdomen and buttock. High energy trauma, long bone fractures, crush or penetrating injury, burns and vascular injury are all predisposing factors. When tissue pressure rises above perfusion pressure, capillary filling is impaired and tissue ischaemia results. Clinical symptoms include severe pain and burning. Sensory loss followed by motor nerve dysfunction may be present on clinical examination.

Measurement of compartment pressure should be undertaken if compartment syndrome is considered. Debate exists regarding the threshold pressure at which to perform fasciotomy but above 30 mmHg is recommended by many. Early fasciotomy (within 6 hours) following the onset of compartment syndrome can be limb saving. If fasciotomy is delayed, permanent nerve damage, loss of limb and death can result.

3

Question 11

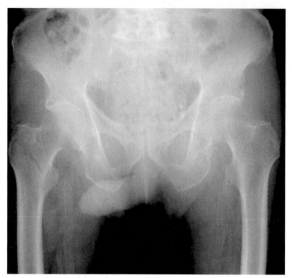

- What type of fracture (Fig. 3.39) is this?

- How does the classification of hip fractures related to healing?

- What are the main causes of morbidity and mortality following hip fracture?

Fig. 3.39 Quiz case.

Answer

Intertrochanteric fracture of the hip

Hip fracture classification
1. Femoral head fractures

2. Femoral neck fractures (Fig. 3.40)

3. Intertrochanteric fractures

4. Trochanteric fractures

5. Subtrochanteric fractures

The anatomical site of a fracture has a significant impact on healing. Femoral head and femoral neck fractures are both intracapsular, whereas intertrochanteric, trochanteric and subtrochanteric fractures are extracapsular. Intracapsular fractures are more prone to complications of healing such as avascular necrosis.

This is consequence of the critical blood supply to the region. Blood supply is derived from three main sources which include

- perforating branches of medial and lateral circumflex artery,

- inferior and superior gluteal arteries,

- obturator artery (posterior branch).

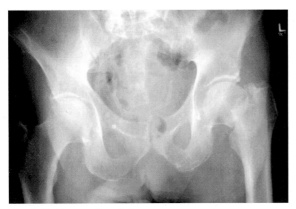

Fig. 3.40 Femoral neck fracture.

In the majority of people the foveal artery which runs with the ligamentum teres to reach the femoral head is insufficient to supply the entire femoral head.

Femoral neck fractures especially if displaced frequently lead to avascular necrosis of the femoral head due to disruption of the interosseus and capsular vessels (which run with the periosteum of the femoral neck).

Mortality and morbidity associated with hip fractures is considerable. Mortality is greatest in the elderly, is highest in the first few months but remains high for up to 1 year afterwards. The immediate mortality after repair of fractured neck of femur is less when spinal anaesthesia is used rather than a general anaesthetic, probably because of a reduction in thromboembolic complications. However, at 1 month there is no difference in outcome between the two techniques.

Morbidity due to surgery and anaesthesia:

- Mal/non-union

- Infection

- Pneumonia

- DVT and pulmonary embolism

- Muscle wasting

The problems following fractured neck of femur are closely linked to immobilisation. In the months following hip fracture reduced ambulation and mobility leads to a loss of independence, reduced quality of life and often depression in the elderly.

Reference
1. Advanced Trauma Life Program for Doctors, 6th edn. American College of Surgeons, Chicago, 1997.

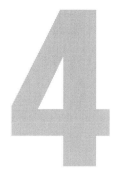

The cervical spine

Savvas Nicolaou, Richard Gee, Lai Peng Chan,
Cieran Keogh, Peter Munk

Introduction: clearing the cervical spine

The cervical spine has been traditionally divided into an upper segment (skull base, C1 and C2), and a lower segment comprising C3–C7. This is not arbitrary and is actually based on specific embryological, morphological and physiologically distinct differences. The characteristics of these two segments become particularly relevant when considering the effects of traumatic events. The most common level is C2 which accounts for 24% of fractures.

The cervical spine attains an importance to the anaesthetist as proper head position is important for successful orotracheal intubation. The oral, pharyngeal and laryngeal axes must be aligned for direct laryngoscopy. The head needs to be elevated at least 10 cm above the shoulders to align the pharyngeal and laryngeal axes. Also the atlanto-occipital joint needs to be extended to achieve the straightest possible line from the incisors to the glottis [1]. A difficult airway is characterised by a limited range of motion at the cervical spine or temporomandibular joint. It can be encountered in conditions such as diffuse idiopathic skeletal hyperostosis (DISH), ankylosing spondylitis, rheumatoid arthritis, juvenile chronic arthritis, Klippel-Feil syndrome (congenital fusion of upper cervical segment) and in the presence of suspected or unknown spinal injury (fracture) in which orotracheal intubation might be contraindicated.

The examination

There is diversity of opinion regarding the initial imaging of a patient suspected of having a cervical spine injury. It is generally accepted that patients with suspected acute cervical spine injury are initially evaluated using plain film radiography. The minimum should include at least three projections: an anteroposterior (AP) view, a lateral view and an open mouth odontoid view [2]. Depending on the clinical scenario and physical condition of the patient, other useful plain film projections include oblique views which might add visualisation of the neuroforamina, facet joints and in a trauma situation they might be extremely helpful in visualising the posterolateral aspects of the lower cervical and upper thoracic vertebrae. Secondly, a swimmer's view in a trauma situation might also be helpful. This is usually obtained with one arm extended above the head and one by the side and helps to visualise the C7/T1 junction. Thirdly, flexion–extension views might be helpful, where atlanto-axial subluxation is a possibility or ligamentous damage is suspected and is usually done in trauma situations when the patient is in severe pain but the initial radiographs appear normal. This must be done under close medical supervision. The patient must control the movement himself or herself as muscle guarding will help prevent an injury.

In most trauma cases, the cervical spine may be cleared by excellent complete lateral visualisation of the cervical spine, open mouth odontoid view and AP views at the risk of missing significant fractures in fewer than 1% of cervical spinal injuries [3].

Depending on the clinical scenario, cervical computed tomography may be used as a screening examination (patients with neurological deficit, severe head injury, high-risk mechanism, unconscious, multi-injured patient), or as a complementary technique to radiography. Usually, magnetic resonance imaging (MRI) is indicated in all patients with partial or progressive neurological deficit after cervical spinal injury and in patients with potential mechanical instability caused by ligamentous injury or associated disc space injury.

In trauma situations, the examination of the cervical spine must cover the area from the base of the skull through the seventh cervical segment. If the cervicothoracic junction is not completely visualised by plain film radiograph, then this needs to be cleared by computed tomography (Figs 4.1 and 4.2).

The quality of the radiographic examination is extremely important. It must be of optimum technical quality to demonstrate both soft tissue and bony anatomy.

4

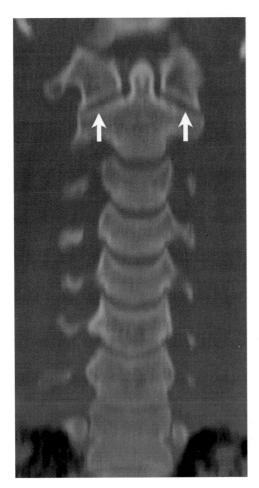

Fig. 4.1 Normal cervical spine. Coronal CT reconstruction. Normal relationship of C1 lateral masses to articular facets of C2 shown with arrows.

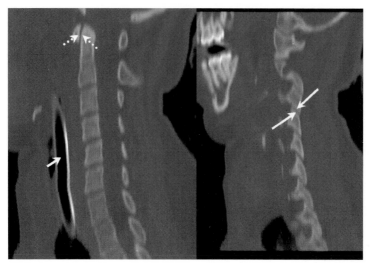

Fig. 4.2 Normal cervical spine. Sagittal CT reformats. Endotracheal tube (solid white arrow) and normal atlantodens interval (dotted arrows) with normal vertebral body alignment. Normal facets demonstrated (long white solid arrows).

General statements: plain film radiography

The lateral radiograph (Fig. 4.3) is the single most important component in the radiographic assessment of the acutely injured cervical spine. Proper patient positioning is essential in obtaining a true lateral radiograph. The degree of laterallarity is assessed usually by the superimposition of the paired articular masses (Fig. 4.4). Usually, the degree of rotation of the head is indicated by

1. lack of superimposition of the angles of the mandible,

2. the articular masses and facet joints becoming superimposed upon the vertebral bodies, and lack of superimposition of the facet joints resulting in a 'bat-wing' or 'bow-tie' appearance.

If the entire body is rotated, there is usually a uniform distance between the posterior cortical margins of the articular masses at each level. If the head is rotated, there is usually a greater distance between the posterior margins of the articular masses and a concomitant decrease in the lamina space. This can be differentiated from a unilateral interfacet dislocation in which there is usually a component of both flexion and rotation [2]. Thus, on top of the rotation, there is usually anterior translation of one vertebral segment relative to another by more than 4 mm indicating the flexion component of the injury.

AP radiograph of the cervical spine (Fig. 4.5) usually visualises the cervical spine from C3 to the upper thoracic segments. It provides valuable evidence of flexion injuries such as anterosubluxation, lateral interfacet dislocation, clay shoveler's fracture (see Question 13) and burst fractures of

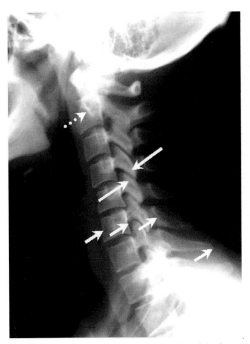

Fig. 4.3 Normal lateral radiograph. This demonstrates all seven cervical vertebrae, down to the cervicothoracic junction. There is normal alignment of vertebral bodies, spinolaminar line and interspinous distances. In particular, the prevertebral soft tissue thickness in the retropharyngeal (anterior to C2) and retrotracheal (anterior to C6) regions is normal. Facet joints are demonstrated with long solid white arrows. Solid short arrows point to normal anterior vertebral line, posterior vertebral line, spinolaminar line, and posterior spinous process line to be intact. Projecting over the C2 body is the sclerotic ring known as the Harris ring (dotted arrow), and this is intact. If disrupted, this is suggestive of a type 3 odontoid fracture.

the lower cervical spine. Frontal projection is the only plain film study in which the uncovertebral body process fracture can be identified [4].

The open mouth projection (Fig. 4.6) is designed to demonstrate the atlanto-axial relationship in the AP projection. It is valuable in recognising fractures of the lateral mass of C1, a Jefferson burst fracture (see Question 7), high- and low-dens fractures, atlanto-axial rotary subluxation/dislocation.

Occasionally, oblique views are helpful in demonstrating not only the intervertebral foramen and facet joint alignment, but also provides additional views of the cervicothroacic junction for alignment [2] (Fig. 4.7).

Normal cervical spine

After assessing that the lateral radiograph is a true lateral, the following lines should always be checked.

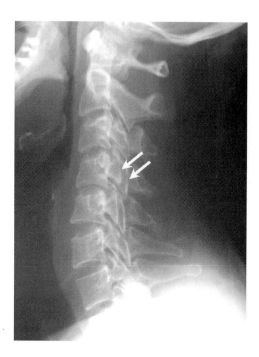

Fig. 4.4 Rotated lateral radiograph. Lack of superimposition of the articular masses, giving the appearance of double articular facets (arrows).

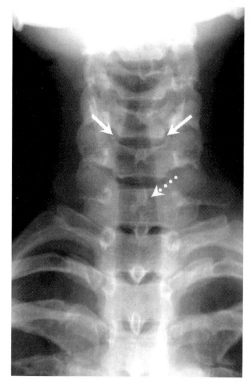

Fig. 4.5 Normal AP radiograph. The AP view usually only demonstrates C3–C7. The uncovertebral joints (arrows) and spinous processes (dotted arrows) can be evaluated. Note the equidistance between the spinous processes.

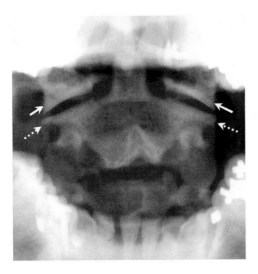

Fig. 4.6 Normal odontoid process view or 'Open mouth' peg view. This view best evaluates the alignment of the lateral masses of C1 (arrows) on the articular pillars of C2 (dotted arrows), the space on either side of the dens with respect to the C1 lateral masses (lateral atlantodens interval), and the odontoid process (dens).

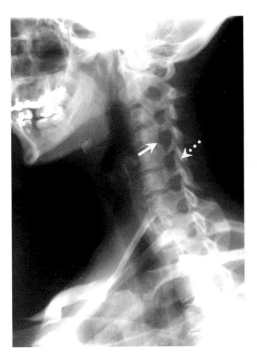

Fig. 4.7 Oblique view of cervical spine. This is helpful in demonstrating not only the intervertebral foramen (arrow) and facet joint alignment (dotted arrow), but also provides additional views of the cervicothoracic junction for alignment.

Soft tissue contour

Position of the normal contour of the prevertebral soft tissue shadow along both the cervical cranium and cervical thoracic junction is extremely important (Fig. 4.8). The cervical cranial prevertebral soft tissue contour should follow the contour of the anterior cortex of the atlas, axis and caudal portion of the clivus. At the cervical thoracic junction, the normal

169

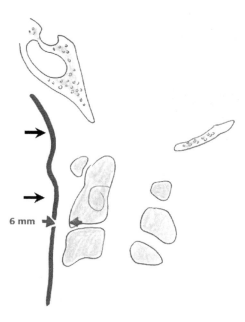

Fig. 4.8 Normal cervical cranial prevertebral soft tissue contour. Cranio cervical prevertebral soft tissue contour (black line between arrow levels) should have a concave, convex (over C1 anterior arch) and concave contour. A measurement of more than 5–7 mm at the C2 level is abnormal, and anterior to vertebra C4–C7 less than 20–22 mm.

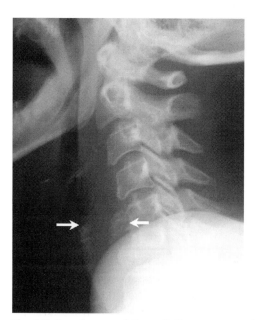

Fig. 4.9 Prominence of the soft tissue contour. Cervical spine osteomyelitis, with prevertebral abscess. Lateral cervical spine. This lateral cervical-spine radiograph shows marked widening of the lower prevertebral soft tissues (arrows) anterior to the C5 level with bony destruction of the C4 vertebral body. This was due to prevertebral abscess in association with cervical osteomyelitis. Gas can sometimes migrate into this potential space from aerodigestive tract injuries. Haemorrhage identified here may be the most prominent radiographic sign of a subtle cervical-spine fracture.

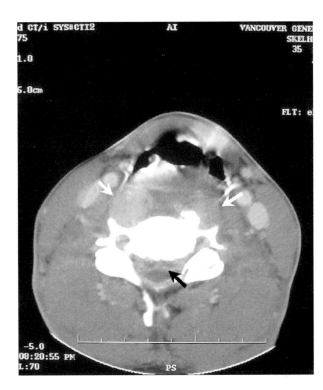

Fig. 4.10 Transverse CT image with IV contrast. The CT image shows a large prevertebral abscess (white arrows) from C5 osteomyelitis. An epidural abscess component is also present encroaching on the thecal sac (black arrow).

contour of the prevertebral soft tissue should also follow the contour of the anterior cortex of the lower cervical vertebral bodies and demonstrate no convexity as it dips and tucks into the thoracic inlet [2, 4]. Prominence of the soft tissue contour may indicate haemorrhage, which can be the most prominent radiographic sign of subtle cervical-spine fracture (Figs 4.9 and 4.10). Various measurements have been described in the literature regarding prevertebral soft tissue thickness. However, the most reliable is the cervical soft tissue thickness present anterior to the cortex of the body of C2 [2] while the remainder are usually unreliable and variable. Anterior to vertebra C2, the distance should be less than 6 mm, and anterior to vertebra C4–C7 less than 20–22 mm.

Clearing the craniocervical junction

The atlantodental interval (Fig. 4.11) normally is less than 3 mm in adults whether or not the head is flexed or extended. In children under 8 years of age, the distance has been reported to be as much as 4–5 mm (particularly in flexion) secondary to the greater ligamentous laxity [5].

Anterior pseudosubluxation (physiological subluxation) of C2 on C3 or C3 on C4 is a normal finding on the lateral cervical spine in children (usually under 8 years of age or young adults) and is due to greater ligamentous laxity. This is caused by the relative laxity of the ligaments combined with the shallow facet joints seen in these young adults. To distinguish it from true subluxation, one must draw a line from

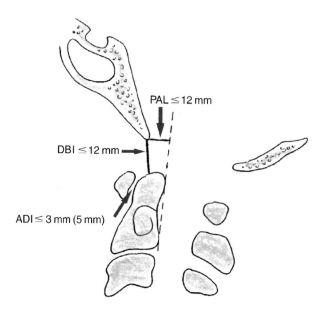

PAL ≤ 12 mm

DBI ≤ 12 mm

ADI ≤ 3 mm (5 mm)

Fig. 4.11 The atlantodental interval ADI normally is less than 3 mm in adults whether or not the head is flexed or extended. In children under 8-years of age, the distance has been reported to be as much as 4–5 mm. Normal measurements ADI (anterior dens interval) ≤3 mm. DBI (dens basion interval) ≤12 mm. PAL (posterior axial line) ≤12 mm.

the spinal lamina of C1 to the spinal lamina of C3 [Fig. 4.12]. This is known as the posterocervical line and it establishes that the apparent subluxation is physiological. Usually, the spinal lamina line of C2 should not be offset by more than 1 mm from the posterocervical line. The radiographic absence of this posterospinal lamina line usually at C1 reflects incomplete fusion of the posterior arches, which is relatively common and precludes use of the C1/C3 spinal lamina relationships discussed. In older people, there may be osteophytic extension beyond this line, and this may be ignored.

The best means of detecting subtle displacements at the craniocervical junction (dislocation/subluxations) is usually the measurement of the shortest distance between the dens and the basion, and the shortest distance between the posterior axial line (PAL) and the basion, not exceeding 12 mm [2] (Fig. 4.13).

Important caveat

Large precervical haematoma is a common finding amongst serious maxillofacial fractures (Le Fort spectrum) [4]. This should be considered when an abnormal cervical cranium prevertebral soft tissue thickening is identified, and precludes using the prevertebral soft tissue interface prominence as a means of identifying cervical-spine fractures.

Open mouth AP radiograph

Usually, on the neutral AP open mouth radiograph, the margin of the atlas and the axis are aligned. The distance between the peg and the lateral masses of C1 should also be equal. Lateral translation of C1 on C2 is normally less than 2 mm. Side-to-side difference in the lateral atlatodens interval exceeding 2 mm is considered abnormal [4] (Fig. 4.14).

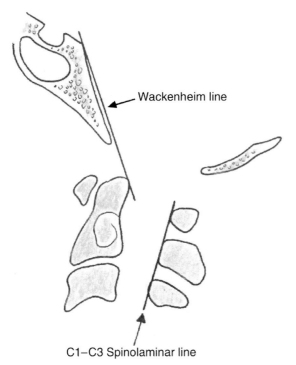

Wackenheim line

C1–C3 Spinolaminar line

Fig. 4.12 Diagram of C1–C3 spinolaminar line, and Wackenheim's line. Spinolaminar line intact. Wackenheim clivus line should intersect the posterior aspect of the odontoid process, however this is not as reliable as the DBI or PAL line in assessing for occipito-atlantal dissociation, given that this line can vary with the steepness of the clivus, or the angulation of the odontoid process.

4

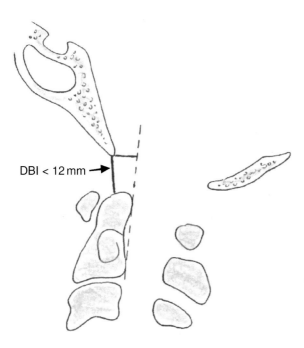

DBI < 12 mm

Fig. 4.13 Craniocervical dissociation. The DBI is normal if less than 12 mm. When the interval is greater than 12 mm, this indicates craniocervical dissociation.

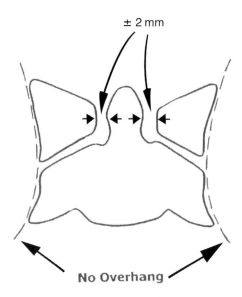

± 2 mm

No Overhang

Fig. 4.14 Diagram of AP peg view. This diagram demonstrates the LDI (lateral dens interval) which should be symmetric. This can be asymmetric, due to rotation. No 'overhang' of the C1 lateral masses should be present.

It is important to remember the sclerotic ring (Harris ring) that is usually seen to project over the C2 vertebral body represents superimposition of the pedicles of C2. When this is disrupted, it signifies a type 3 odontoid fracture (fracture of the body of C2), and can be the only clue in revealing a type 3 fracture. This can be deficient posteriorly and inferiorly due to the superimposition of the foramina transversarium of C2 [2].

Additional lines to be checked on the lateral radiograph (Fig. 4.15) include the anterior and posterior margins of the vertebral bodies known as the anterior and posterior vertebral body lines. These should be gently curved and continuous. Thirdly, the spinal lamina line is drawn along longitudinally through the sclerotic line at the junction of the spinous process with the lamina and should also form a smooth continuous arc. The exception to this rule is that there may be a slight step of less than 2 mm in the spinous process arc, especially in children. A step greater than 2 mm is abnormal and may indicate a fracture or dislocation. Fourthly, a continuous concave line should follow along the tips of the spinous processes. Usually disruption of the anterovertebral line can be seen in anterior subluxations that is normally seen with cervical degenerative joint disease change. Anterior listhesis of 2–3 mm is usually seen in severe degenerative disc disease and if more than 3 mm, it needs to be further evaluated depending on the clinical scenario with either flexion/extension views or a CT scan.

AP view
The spinous process should lie in a straight line (remembering that there are bifid spinous processes within the cervical spine), and must be approximately equidistant from the levels above and below. If this is not the case, it is suggestive of a unilateral or bilateral facet joint dislocation.

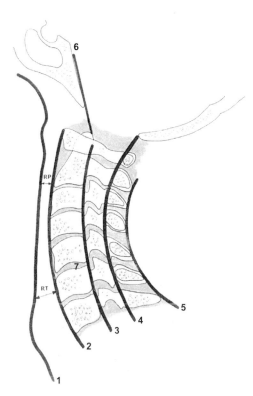

Fig. 4.15 Normal alignment lines: 1. Prevertebral soft tissue line, 2. anterior vertebral body line, 3. posterior vertebral body line, 4. spinolaminar line, 5. interspinous process line, 6. clivus to dens line (Wackenheim line), 7. disc space height. The interval between lines 3 and 4 represents the spinal canal. RP = retropharyngeal soft tissue thickness (anterior to C2) – normal = less than 6 mm. RT = retrotracheal soft tissue thickness (anterior to C6) – normal = less than 21 mm.

Special caveats
The lateral view of the upper cervical spine and lower part of the skull is important in evaluating (vertical subluxation) vertical superior migration of the odontoid process into the foramen magnum. There are certain measurements that are helpful in determining atlanto-axial migration/cranial settling or vertical migration of the odontoid process (terms that are often used interchangeably) (Fig. 4.16). This condition can be seen in rheumatoid arthritis, trauma, Paget's disease and congenital conditions such as Down's syndrome [6].

Second caveat
Stenosis on a lateral radiograph can be inferred if the AP dimension of the canal measures less than 16 mm at C1/C2 or usually less than 13 mm from C3 through to C7 (see Fig. 4.15). However, canal stenosis is most accurately assessed on CT and MRI, and MRI can also display intrinsic cord abnormalities [6].

Injury to the cervical spine
One of the most important questions in suspected cervical injury is the question of stability of a fracture or a dislocation. Stability of the vertebral column usually depends on the integrity of the major skeletal components, discs, apophyseal joints and ligamentous structures. Radiographic findings

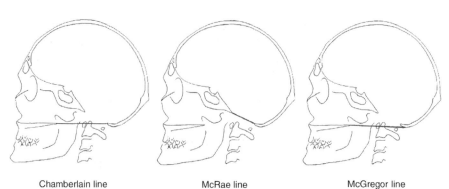

| Chamberlain line | McRae line | McGregor line |

Fig. 4.16 Atlanto-axial impaction cranial settling. *Chamberlain line*: Posterior margin of hard palate to posterior margin of foramen magnum (opisthion). Normal = tip of dens up to 3 mm above this line. *McRae line*: anterior margin of foramen magnum (basion) to posterior margin of foramen magnum (opisthion). Normal = dens below this line. A perpendicular line from the apex of dens should cross the McRae line in the anterior quarter. *McGregor line*: posterosuperior margin of hard palate to most caudal part of occipital curve of skill. normal = dens tip up to 5 mm above this line. In studies, the most reliable and practical line is the McRae line.

that indicate instability according to Daffner [7] are displacement of vertebrae greater than 4 mm, widening of the interspinous or interlamina spaces, widening of the apophyseal joints, widening and elongation of the vertebral canal, widening of the interpedicular distance in the transverse and vertical planes, and disruption of the posterovertebral body line. Only one of these features needs to be present to make a radiographic assumption of an unstable injury.

> The cervical spine can be cleared clinically only in the fully conscious, unintoxicated and cooperative patient in whom there is no neck pain, no bony tenderness, no abnormal neurology, no distracting injuries and pain free full range of neck movements.

> Mechanisms of cervical spinal trauma are hyperflexion, hyperextension and compression. Usually, the six cervical spine injuries considered to be unstable are bilateral locked facets, type 2 odontoid fractures, flexion teardrop fracture, hangman's fracture (depending on degree of displacement), Jefferson's fracture, and a burst fracture with involvement of the posterior elements, or associated compression fracture of more than 25% of the affected vertebral body.

Clearing the cervical spine in the unconscious/obtunded patient
There is no clear consensus on the best way to clear the cervical spine in victims of blunt trauma with altered mental status. Plain radiography may not detect injury to ligaments and some of these may be significant, unstable injuries. There are problems associated with maintaining cervical immobilisation in the unconscious patient for a prolonged period.

4

The hard collar can cause raised intracranial pressure (greater in patients with a head injury) and skin damage and ulceration. Maintenance of the supine position affects drainage of secretion and the need for log-rolling is nurse intensive. The current options are as follows [8]:

1. Leave the cervical spine uncleared and maintain cervical spine stabilisation until the patient is fully awake and can be assessed clinically. The British Trauma Society recommends removing the hard collar but maintaining in-line positioning with sandbags and log-rolling when turning. The collar is then reapplied before the patient is woken up.

2. Review the three cervical radiographs supplemented with thin cut axial CT images with sagittal reconstruction through suspicious or inadequately visualised areas. If these studies are technically adequate and properly interpreted, the false negative rate is 0.1%; many clinicians would then consider the spine stable and remove the immobilisation devices.

3. Assess the stability of the cervical spine by flexion/extension fluoroscopy. Not all physicians consider dynamic fluoroscopy to be safe in unconscious patients. This should only be done in consultation with senior consultants experienced in the management of spinal injuries.

4. Obtain magnetic resonance (MR) scans of the cervical spine. This may reveal ligament injury without the need to stress the spine but it is expensive and technically difficult in patients undergoing invasive monitoring or who are too ill to be in the scanner for a long time.

These options are summarised in Table 4.1.

Summary

Recall evaluation of the lateral cervical spine film in trauma (Fig. 4.15)
Countdown to T1; all seven cervical vertebrae should be well seen.
Evaluate the thickness of the retropharyngeal/retrotracheal space.
Less than 5–7 mm anterior to the vertebra at C1/C3 and less than 20–22 mm anterior to the vertebra C4–C7.

Assess the four parallel lines for incongruity
The four parallel lines to be assessed for incongruity are anterovertebral line – anterior to the vertebral bodies; posterovertebral line posterior to the vertebral bodies; spinal lamina line; posterior spinous line (tips of the spinous processes).

The atlantodental interval should be evaluated, no more than 3 mm in adults and less than 5 mm in children less than 8 years of age.
If abnormal, suspicious for disruption of the transverse ligament is raised.

Evaluate the disc spaces for narrowing or widening as a result of an acute flexion or extension injury [9].

Table 4.1 Cervical spinal clearance algorithm

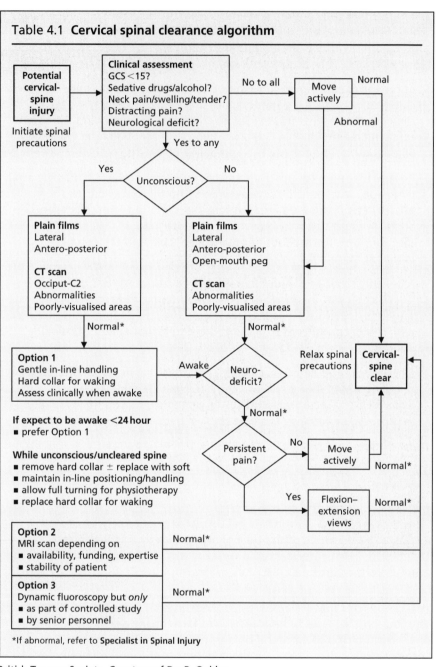

British Trauma Society. Courtesy of Dr. P. Oakley

Non-traumatic conditions affecting the cervical spine

Question 1

74-year-old patient.
History of non-specific neck stiffness (Fig. 4.17) and pain for 3–4 years.

- What is the diagnosis?

- Are there any implications for anaesthesia or intubation?

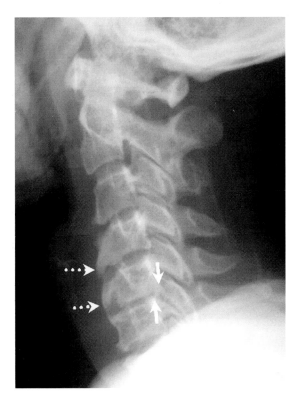

Fig. 4.17 Quiz case.

Answer

Cervical spondylosis

Definitions

- Spondylosis: Non-specific degenerative process of the spine.

- Spondylolisthesis: Anterior subluxation of one vertebral body on another.

- Spondylolysis: Failure of the neural arch manifesting as a defect in the pars interarticularis [6].

Degenerative changes may involve the spine as osteoarthritis of the synovial joints resulting in subchondral sclerosis, osteophyte formation and joint space narrowing. Degenerative disc disease manifest as disc space narrowing, discogenic sclerosis, vacuum disc phenomenon and associated anterior and posterior end-plate osteophyte formation. Osteophyte formation may also encroach the neural foramina (resulting in stenoses) leading to radicular symptoms.

Degenerative changes may also involve the fibrous articulations, tendons or sets of ligaments attached to the bones leading to a condition known as DISH [5].

The complications of degenerative joint disease to the spine are usually degenerative spondylolisthesis or spinal stenosis.

The clinical significance is that these changes may result in limited mobility making an intubation difficult. They may also result in spinal claudication, cervical myelopathy or radiculopathy. Stenosis of the spine may take the form of central spinal canal stenosis, stenosis of the lateral recess or narrowing of the neural foramina. Evaluation of spinal stenosis from plain film radiography has been mentioned in the beginning of this chapter. Spinal stenosis can be better assessed using computed tomography or MRI, if indicated clinically.

The most common level of the cervical spine to be involved by cervical spondylosis is the C5/C6 disc space level, and is most commonly seen in middle-aged people and beyond.

Question 2

- How may this condition (Figs 4.18–4.20) affect intubation?
- What are the other manifestations of this condition?

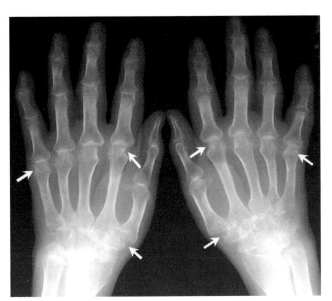

Fig. 4.18 Quiz case.

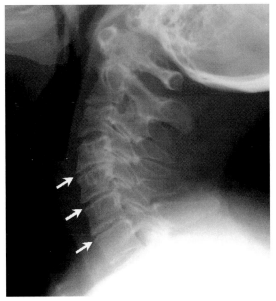

Fig. 4.19 Quiz case.

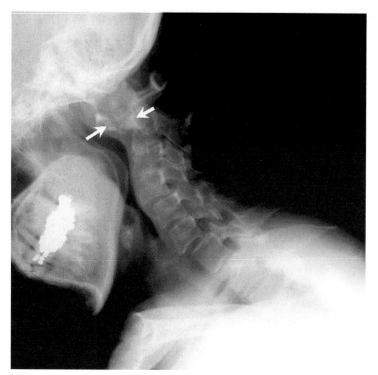

Fig. 4.20 Quiz case.

Answer

Craniocervical junction and cervical spine abnormalities

Certain conditions that affect the craniocervical junction and cervical spine are clinically relevant to anaesthetists. These conditions can result in difficult endotracheal intubation, owing to limited mobility of the head and neck. Inability to extend the head and flex the neck (sniffing position) can prevent the anaesthetist from achieving the ideal position for direct visualisation of the glottic opening which requires alignment of the three axes, i.e. the mouth, pharynx and trachea.

Rheumatoid arthritis

Rheumatoid arthritis is a progressive chronic systemic inflammatory disorder affecting primarily the synovial joints. Women are three times more commonly affected than men. Characteristically, it is a symmetrical inflammatory arthropathy affecting peripheral small joints, i.e. hands and feet, which may also affect larger joints (hips, knees and elbows).

It usually commences with progressive pain, stiffness and joint swelling. Early findings include periarticular soft tissue and tendon sheath swelling. Deformities include the swan-neck and boutonniere deformities, ulna deviation at the MCP joints and carpal drift in volar and palmar directions.

Bony changes include symmetric narrowing of the joint space associated with marginal or central erosions and periarticular osteopenia. Subchondral sclerosis is minimal or absent and formation of osteophytes is usually lacking unless end-stage disease is present. The usual joints that are affected are the MCP joints, the radial and ulnar styloid processes, distal radial ulna joints, and the carpus where ankylosis or bony resorption and erosions may occur.

More than 80% of patients with moderate to severe rheumatoid arthritis have radiographic evidence of cervical-spine involvement (Figs 4.19 and 4.20). Do not assume the cervical spine is normal. The most characteristic radiographic findings involve the odontoid process, atlanto-axial joint and apophyseal joints of the subaxial spine. The erosive changes usually affect the odontoid process resulting in loosening the insertion of the transverse ligament of the atlas. This leads to instability allowing anterior subluxation of the atlas on the axis. This may result in cervical spinal cord compression. This is frequently accompanied by a vertical translocation of the odontoid process, also known as cranial settling or basilar impression (depending on which literature you read). The laxity of the transverse ligament is usually apparent on the lateral radiograph. The findings are accentuated by flexion when there is a marked increase in the atlantodental interval. It often requires surgical intervention with the usual procedure being a posterior fusion [5, 6].

Atlanto-axial subluxation in rheumatoid arthritis is usually progressive and the greater the degree of myelopathy, the higher the risk of sudden death. The end result of vertical migration of the odontoid process (cranial settling) leads to compression of the pons and medulla. Rheumatoid granulation (inflammatory panus) behind the odontoid also contributes to this effect and vertebral artery obstruction may also play a role. The degree of erosion of C1 usually correlates with the extent of superior migration of the odontoid process [6].

MRI is the best test to evaluate the compression of the upper cord and pons/medulla as this best demonstrates the location of the odontoid process, extent of inflammatory pannus, and associated edematous changes to the spinal cord [6] (Figs 4.21 and 4.22). Commonly, rheumatoid arthritis may affect the apophyseal joints or disc spaces in the subaxial cervical spine, further changes include subluxation, bone destruction or even ankylosis. If the discs are involved, there may be erosion or even fusion.

Pulmonary manifestations include unilateral pleural effusions, pulmonary fibrosis (Figs 4.23 and 4.24) affecting the lower lobes, rheumatoid nodules which may be single or multiple and are commonly subpleural in location. Caplan's syndrome is rheumatoid nodules in the lungs of coal miners with silicosis. The most common early manifestation is bronchiolitis obliterans (respiratory bronchiolar inflammation with air trapping/mosaic perfusion, bronchiectasis) [10]. This is usually identified on high-resolution CT scans with expiratory views. Pulmonary complications in rheumatoid arthritis are most commonly seen in men with seropositive disease.

The anaesthetist should always assess neck movement in patients with rheumatoid arthritis. Recent flexion/extension neck views or MRI should be examined for evidence of the separation of the odontoid peg from the atlas, or subluxation of cervical vertebrae. If the neck is unstable, the case should be managed by a consultant anaesthetist. If the patient has temperomandibular joint involvement reducing mouth opening, then the airway management becomes even more problematical. Regional techniques should always be considered. If intubation is required, then awake fibre-optic intubation may be used. If the neck is unstable, a hard collar and sandbags should be used while the patient is unconscious to prevent neck movement.

4

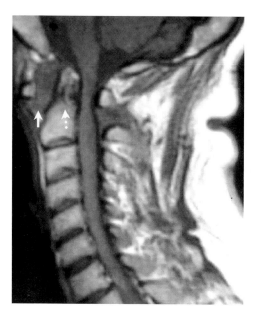

Fig. 4.21 MRI (T1) of cervical spine in rheumatoid arthritis. There is added tissue of intermediate signal (arrows) between the dens and anterior arch of C1, with widening of the anterior atlanto-axial interval, with erosion of the dens (dotted arrow) and compression on the spinal cord.

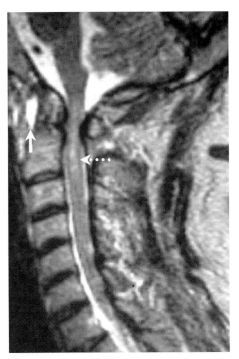

Fig. 4.22 MRI (T2) of cervical spine in rheumatoid arthritis. Images show high-signal material anterior (arrow) to the odontoid process. This indicates an inflammatory pannus. Pannus can also be present around the attachments of the transverse and cruciate ligaments. MRI is also useful for showing degree of compression on the cervical cord, and also demonstrates increased signal within the cord, due to cervical myelopathy (dotted arrow).

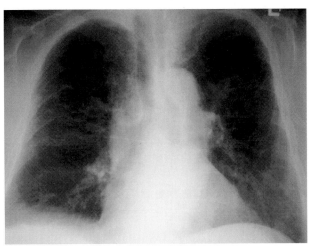

Fig. 4.23 Rheumatoid arthritis. Lung manifestations chest X-ray – basal fibrosis.

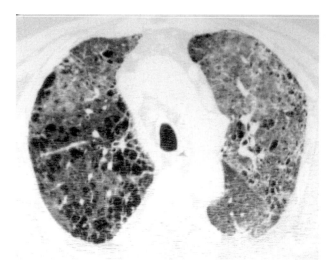

Fig. 4.24 Rheumatoid arthritis. Lung manifestations. There is extensive end-stage pulmonary fibrosis (honeycombing), with thickened interlobular septae, ground glass density (representing activity of disease) due to rheumatoid lung.

4

Question 3

23-year-old female patient with a chronic rheumatological condition
(Figs 4.25–4.27).

■ What are the features which will affect anaesthetic management?

■ What is the condition?

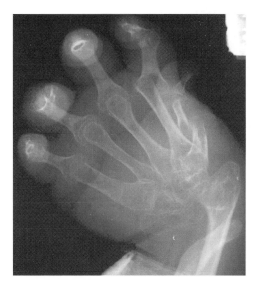

Fig. 4.25 Quiz case.

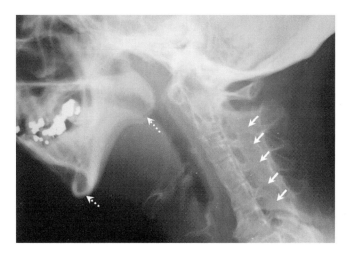

Fig. 4.26 Quiz case.

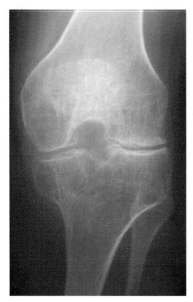 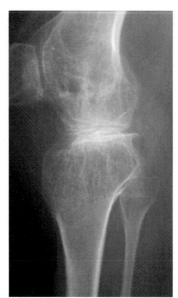

Fig. 4.27 Quiz case.

4

Answer

Juvenile rheumatoid arthritis

Juvenile rheumatoid arthritis (JRA) is a chronic inflammatory synovial disease usually affecting children. Girls are more frequently affected than boys. This disease exhibits many of the features of adult rheumatoid arthritis. There are three additional features that are almost pathognomonic of this condition, if these are present. First is periosteal reaction that is usually seen along the shafts of the proximal phalanges and metacarpals, next is joint ankylosis that may occur not only in the wrist but also in the interphalangeal articulations (Fig. 4.25). Fusion of the apophyseal joints of the cervical spine is a characteristic finding (Fig. 4.26), in addition to fusion of the posterior elements. The last of the pathognomonic features is growth abnormality. Altered bone growth is a common finding because the onset of JRA usually occurs before the closure of the growth plates. Involvement of the epiphyseal regions often leads to fusion of the growth plates with resultant retardation of bone growth. Paradoxically, this might also precipitate premature acceleration of growth due to stimulation of the growth plate by resultant hyperemia. The enlargement of the epiphyses of the distal femur usually leads to characteristic overgrowth of the condyles in the knee [5] (Fig. 4.27).

The implication for anesthesia is that there is limited mobility of the spine due to the bony ankylosis, and there is usually micrognathia due to the growth disturbance. These factors can make intubation extremely difficult.

Question 4

46-year-old male patient.

Haematemesis requiring central line insertion and resuscitation.

■ What is the condition (Figs 4.28–4.31)?

■ What are the implications for the anaesthetist?

■ What may have precipitated the haematemesis?

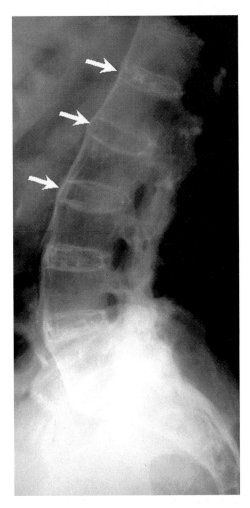

Fig. 4.28 Quiz case.

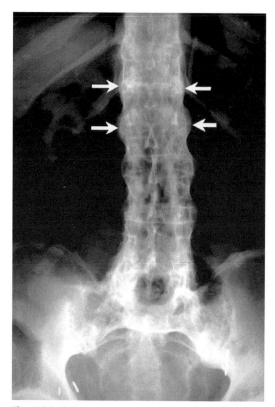

Fig. 4.29 Quiz case.

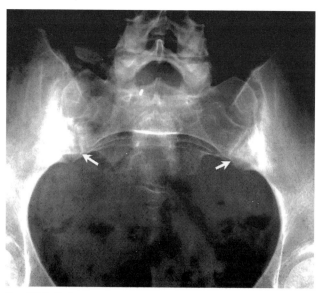

Fig. 4.30 Quiz case.

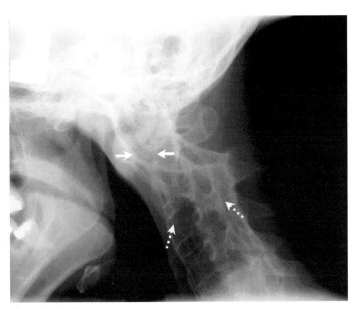

Fig. 4.31 Quiz case.

Answer

Ankylosing spondylitis

Ankylosing spondylitis is a chronic progressive inflammatory arthritis principally affecting the synovial joints of the spine and adjacent soft tissues, as well as the sacro-iliac joints. Peripheral joints such as the hips, shoulders and knees may also be involved. It usually presents in young men and women, being seven times more frequently seen in men with an insidious onset of lower back pain and stiffness. There is an extremely strong link to the antigen HLA-B27, with approximately 97% of patients being positive for this antigen. These patients do exhibit extra-articular features of the disease including iritis, pulmonary fibrosis, cardiac conduction defects, aortic incompetence, spinal cord compression and amyloidosis [5].

Radiographic features

Squaring of the anterior border of the lower thoracic and lumbar vertebrae is one of the earliest radiographic features of ankylosing spondylitis, best demonstrated on the lateral radiograph of the spine (Fig. 4.28). As the condition progresses, delicate desmophytes are formed bridging the vertebral bodies, these have a vertical rather than horizontal orientation distinguishing them from osteophytes of degenerative disease. Paravertebral ossifications are also common. Apophyseal joint and vertebral body fusion usually later on in the course of the disease is a pathognomonic radiographic finding known as the 'bamboo spine' (Fig. 4.29). Sacro-iliac joint involvement is usually present with sacro-iliitis being the hallmark of AS. Most patients will have abnormal sacro-iliac joints radiographically on initial presentation. This is usually a bilateral and symmetric process initially affecting the iliac side of the joint, and progressing along the inferior synovial portion of the joint. The initial signs are osteoporosis, loss of cortical definition, superficial erosions and focal sclerosis with eventual obliteration of the sacro-iliac joint space with resultant bony ankylosis [5] (Fig. 4.30).

Complications of ankylosing spondylitis in the cervical spine include atlanto-axial subluxation (Fig. 4.31), which may become fixed with multilevel spinal fusion. Ankylosing spondylitis patients are more prone to fractures following relatively minor trauma. The fixed spinal segments can result in increased mechanical forces with the formation of a pseudoarthrosis with resultant deformity and bone loss. Ankylosing spondylitis patients are also more predisposed to infection of the spine with tuberculosis.

The implications for anesthesia include difficulties in endotracheal intubation as well as the problems in ventilation associated with a poorly compliant thoracic cage and possibly pulmonary fibrosis affecting the upper lobes. Given the effects on the spine described, this might also affect the application of an epidural anaesthetic.

Long-term use of non-steroidal anti-inflammatory drugs may be complicated by upper gastrointestinal bleeding.

4

Question 5

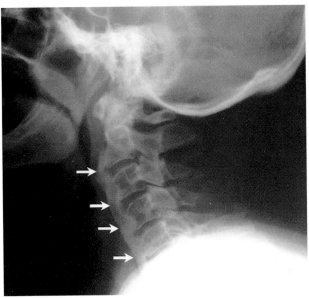

■ What is the diagnosis (Fig. 4.32)?

■ How is it distinguished from ankylosing spondylitis?

Fig. 4.32 Quiz case.

4

Answer

Diffuse idiopathic skeletal hyperostosis

This condition is characterised by flowing ossification along the anterior aspect of the vertebral bodies extending across the disc space. This occurs in the absence of any degenerative, traumatic or postinfectious changes, i.e. the disc space heights are well maintained and there is no disc space loss. It usually affects Caucasians, with a male predominance it is usually seen in patients in their mid-60s.

Most cases occur in the thoracic and lumbar spine (greater than 90% of cases), with the cervical spine involved in greater than 70% of cases (Fig. 4.32). The sacro-iliac joints are spared which can help to differentiate this condition from ankylosing spondylitis.

Patients may have early morning stiffness and mild limitation of activities. They may also present with dysphagia due to compression of the oesophagus between the prominent flowing osteophytes and the rigid laryngeal structures that commonly calcify as people get older.

This condition is associated with hyperostosis at sites of tendon and ligament attachments to the bone, ligamentous ossification and osteophytosis involving the axial and appendicular skeleton [5]. This is best demonstrated on a lateral radiography of the spine (Fig. 4.33).

This condition needs to be distinguished from the previously described 'bamboo spine' seen in ankylosing spondylitis. The sacro-iliac joints are usually spared in DISH, and usually no paravertebral ossification is seen (Fig. 4.34).

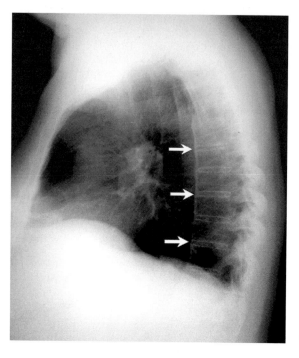

Fig. 4.33 Quiz case.

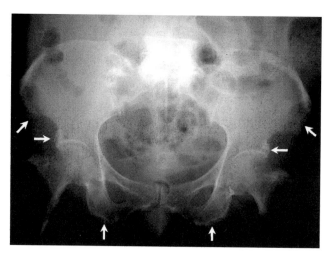

Fig. 4.34 Quiz case.

Trauma of the cervical spine

Airway management in the patient with a suspected cervical spine fracture [8]

Cervical spine injuries occur in 2–5% of blunt trauma patients and of these 7–14% are unstable. All trauma patients should be managed as if they may have a cervical spine injury (Airway with cervical spine control – ATLS guidelines) until the neck is cleared. As long as manual in-line neck stabilisation is applied, rapid sequence induction of anaesthesia, followed by direct laryngoscopy and oral intubation appears to be safe. If intubation is not urgent, an awake fibre-optic intubation is another option.

If intubation of the patient with a potential cervical spine injury fails, or appropriate experienced personnel are unavailable, the laryngeal mask airway or one of its various modifications are alternatives.

4

Question 6

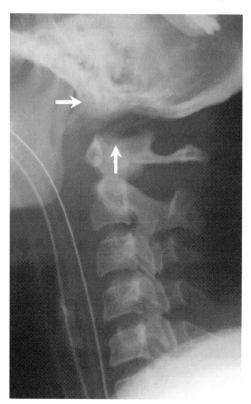

28-year-old male patient. The patient required cardio-pulmonary resuscitation during ambulance transfer to hospital.

■ What is the prognosis (Fig. 4.35)?

Fig. 4.35 Quiz case.

Answer

Occipito-atlantal dissociation

This is a generic term that refers to disruption of the occipito-atlantal articulation that includes partial (subluxation) or complete (dislocation) disruption [2].

Stability of this joint complex is primarily ligamentous. Frank occipito-atlantal dislocation is usually a fatal injury (Fig. 4.35). However, with atlanto-occipital subluxation patients may be neurologically intact. Other forms of presentation are bulbar-cervical dissociation, lower cranial nerve deficits with or without cervical cord injury, or worsening neurological deficit with application of cervical traction.

The diagnosis is easily made by measuring the dens basion interval (DBI) (Fig. 4.13). The distance does not exceed 12 mm in adults or children.

Question 7

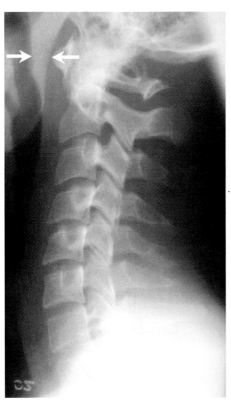

Fig. 4.36 Quiz case.

Male patient. Manual labourer. Struck (whilst wearing protective helmet) on top of head.
Glasgow Coma Score 15/15. Neurologically intact. Complaining of neck pain (Figs 4.36–4.39).

■ What is the injury?

4

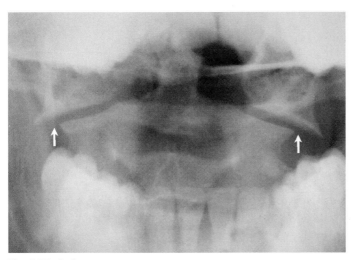

Fig. 4.37 Quiz case.

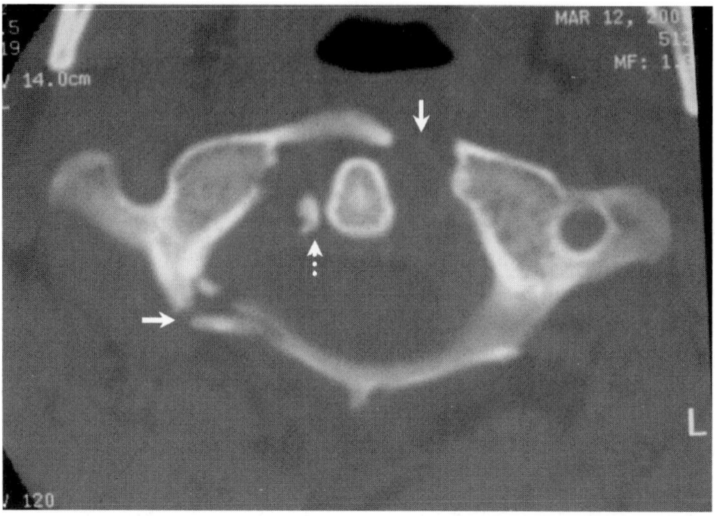

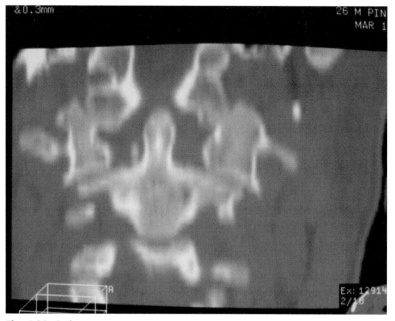

Fig. 4.38 Quiz case.

Fig. 4.39 Quiz case.

Answer

Jefferson fracture

This is usually the result of a vertical compression force ('blow out' fracture). The classic Jefferson fracture involves fractures of both the anterior and posterior arches bilaterally. Usual radiographic features are displacement of the lateral masses of C1 beyond the margins of the body of C2 (Figs 4.36 and 4.37). There is approximately a 41% chance of an associated C2 fracture, thus CT including C1–C3 is recommended [6] (Figs 4.38 and 4.39). One important caveat; the lack of fusion of the posterior arch may be seen in adults as a congenital anomaly defined by smooth margins. This fracture is usually unstable. Usually no neurological deficit is isolated, due to fragments being forced outwards.

Another important caveat is the rule of Spence. On an AP open mouth odontoid view, if the sum total of the overhang of both the C1 lateral masses relative to the body of C2 is greater than or equal to 7 mm, then the inference is that the transverse ligament is probably disrupted (which requires rigid immobilisation).

4

Question 8

Describe the type of fracture (Figs 4.40 and 4.41).

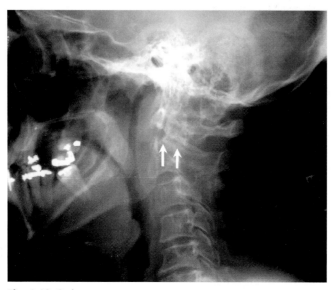

Fig. 4.40 Quiz case.

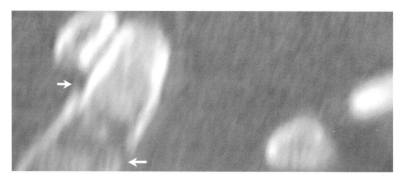

Fig. 4.41 Quiz case.

Answer

Odontoid fracture
There are three types:

■ type 1 – the tip of the odontoid is involved (rare usually stable);

■ type 2 – odontoid fracture is a fracture of the base of the odontoid (unstable ≥ 6 mm displacement) (Figs 4.40 and 4.41);

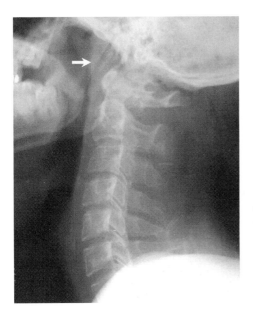

Fig. 4.42 Dens fracture. Lateral cervical spine. A break in the inferior margin of the sclerotic ring found in the body of C2 (Harris' ring), along with prevertebral soft tissue swelling (arrow). This indicates a type 3 dens fracture. This can be the only view where this type of fracture is identified – on the AP odontoid view (Fig. 4.44) the fracture is not visible.

4

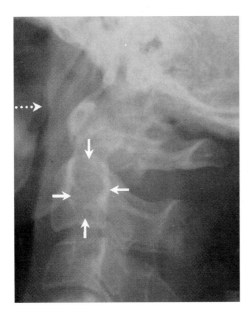

Fig. 4.43 Odontoid fracture (dens fracture). Lateral cervical spine (close up of Fig. 4.42). Disruption of this ring (arrow) may be the only sign of a dens fracture. Soft tissue thickening at C1 level is also present (dotted arrows).

■ type 3 is a fracture through the base of the odontoid that extends through the body of the C2 vertebra.

This is usually a stable injury with a good prognosis, and is identified on the lateral by disruption of Harris' ring [6] (Figs 4.42–4.44).

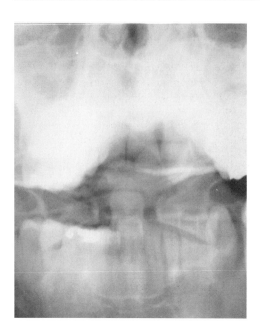

Fig. 4.44 Odontoid (dens fracture). AP peg view. Same patient as Fig. 4.42. A fracture through the body of C2 is not appreciated on the odontoid peg view.

Question 9

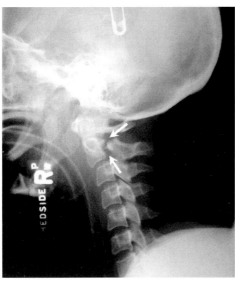

Fig. 4.45 Quiz case.

56-year-old female with long history of depression. Attempted hanging.

- What is this injury called (Figs 4.45 and 4.46)?

4

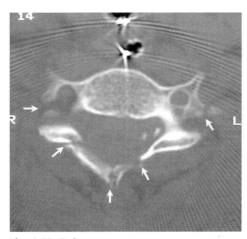

Fig. 4.46 Quiz case.

Answer

Hangman's fracture
This is a traumatic spondylolisthesis of the C2 vertebral body resulting from hyperextension and distraction seen with hanging and from hyperextension and axial loading in motor vehicle accidents when the chin strikes the dashboard.

203

The radiographic features are

- bilateral pars interarticularis fractures of C2 (Figs 4.45 and 4.46),
- anterior dislocation of the C2 vertebral body,
- anterior inferior avulsion fracture associated with the rupture of the anterior longitudinal ligament,
- prevertebral soft tissue swelling (which can be absent at times).

This type of fracture is associated with a high incidence of head injury. The fracture is usually stable, however, instability can be identified by

- marked anterior displacement of C2 on C3 particularly if the degree of displacement exceeds more than 50% of the AP diameter of the C3 vertebral body,
- marked motion on flexion/extension films,
- excessive angulation greater than 11 degrees.

Neurological deficit is rare, non-union is rare and 90% usually heal with immobilisation only [6].

4

Question 10

■ What is the mechanism of this fracture (Figs 4.47 and 4.48)?

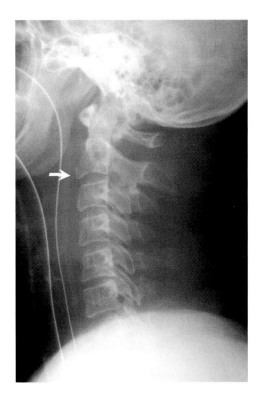

Fig. 4.47 Quiz case.

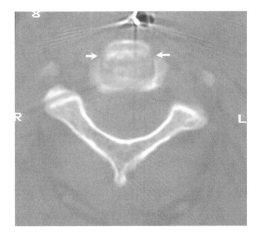

Fig. 4.48 Quiz case.

Answer

Extension teardrop fracture

This is usually the result of a hyperextension injury caused by a force delivered to the face or the mandible that drives the head and neck into an abnormal extension. The extension teardrop fracture is a relatively large triangular fragment with its vertical height equal to or greater than its transverse width. The fractured fragment usually arises from the antero-inferior corner of the involved vertebra, most commonly the C2 vertebral body (Figs 4.47 and 4.48). This is an avulsion fracture at the site of insertion of the intact anterior longitudinal ligament during hyperextension of the head and upper cervical spine. Extension teardrop fractures are more common in older patients with osteopenia and degenerative disease of the spine. This is usually a stable injury in flexion and unstable in extension [2, 6].

Question 11

■ What is the name of this fracture (Figs 4.49–4.51)?

■ What are the radiological features?

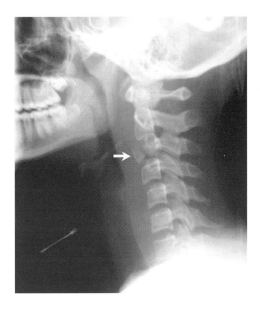

Fig. 4.49 Quiz case.

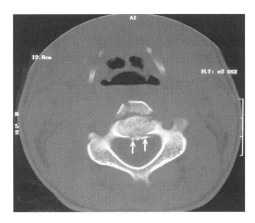

Fig. 4.50 Quiz case.

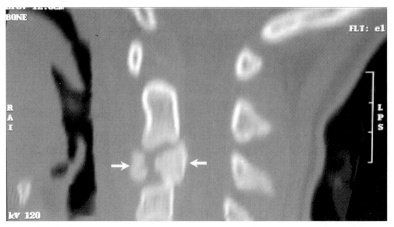

Fig. 4.51 Quiz case.

Answer

Flexion teardrop injury

This usually results from a severe flexion injury that usually occurs with neck injuries caused by diving into shallow water, that results in posterior ligament disruption and an anterior compression fracture of the involved vertebral body. The radiographic features include:

- anterovertebral body avulsion fracture representing the teardrop fragment

- posterovertebral body subluxation or displacement with the disruption of the posterolongitudinal ligament and compromise of the spinal canal with resultant anterior compression of the spinal cord.

Other features include fracture of the spinous process and widening of the interspinous distance due to disruption of the interspinous ligaments, and prevertebral haematoma associated with anterior ligament disruption [2, 5, 8].

This is an unstable injury due to complete disruption of the disc, anterior and posterior ligaments and the facet joints. MRI may help assess the integrity of the disc and ligaments. Patients are often quadriplegic, although some may be neurologically intact.

Question 12

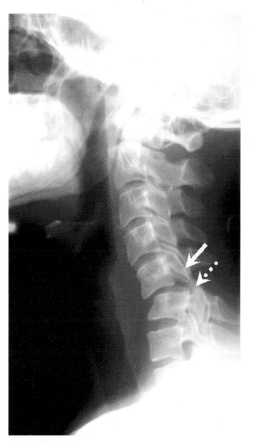

- What is this injury (Fig. 4.52)?

- Is this injury associated with spinal cord damage?

Fig. 4.52 Quiz case.

Answer

Locked facet injuries

This is usually the result of a severe flexion injury which can result in disrupting the normal relationship between the facets. The inferior facet of the level above is usually posterior to the superior facet of the level below. Facets that are just before the point of locking are known as perched facets.

Flexion and rotational injury will result in a unilateral locked facet while an extreme hyperflexion force will result in a bilateral locked facet. Bilateral locked facets usually present with cervical spinal cord injury and injury to the cervical roots.

Diagnosis is usually made on the lateral cervical spine and AP radiographs. Both unilateral and bilateral locked facets will often produce subluxation. Horizontal subluxation of greater than 3.5 mm of

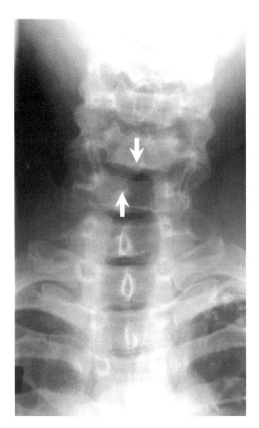

4

Fig. 4.53 Locked facets. AP cervical spine.There is malalignment of the spinous processes (arrows) at the C5–C6 level corresponding to the level of locked facets (Fig. 4.52). Incidental nodular densities and smooth pleural thickening at the left lung apex are calcified granulomas and pleural reaction related to previously healed TB.

one vertebral body on another or greater than 11 degrees of angulation of one vertebral body relative to the next indicates ligamentous instability.

In unilateral facet dislocation, the AP view of the spinous process above the subluxation rotate to the same side as the locked facet (see Fig. 4.53). On the lateral cervical-spine radiograph, 'bow-tie' or 'bat-wing' appearances of the locked facets is seen referring to visualisation of the left and right facets at the level of the injury instead of the usual normal superimposition of the facet joints.

Subluxation may be seen in unilateral locked facets. However, it is almost always seen in bilateral locked facets with usually greater than 25% of the vertebral body being subluxed anterior relative to the vertebral body below. Disruption of the posterior ligamentous complex may produce widening of the interspinous distance and there may also be a widening of the disc space. Oblique films may help better demonstrate the locked facets which usually will be seen blocking the neuroforamina. MRI may be utilised to assess integrity of the disc space and exclude an extruded disc that could be impinging on the spinal cord [2, 5, 6].

Question 13

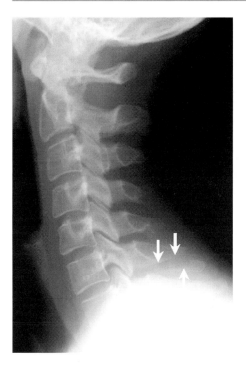

- What is this injury (Figs 4.54 and 4.55)?
- What is the mechanism?
- Is the fracture stable?

Fig. 4.54 Quiz case.

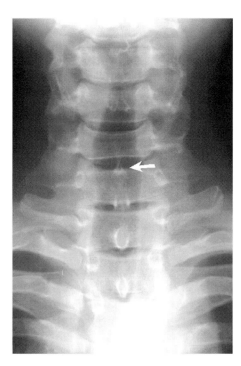

Fig. 4.55 Quiz case.

Answer

Clay Shoveler's fracture

This usually refers to a fracture of the spinous process seen involving the lower cervical spine, usually C7. Initially described in workers who used to shovel clay and during the throwing phase, the clay may stick to the shovel jerking the trapezius or other muscles which are attached to the cervical spinous processes resulting in an avulsion fracture. This fracture may also occur with a whiplash injury or injuries that displace the arms upwards, neck hyperflexion, or a direct blow to the spinous process.

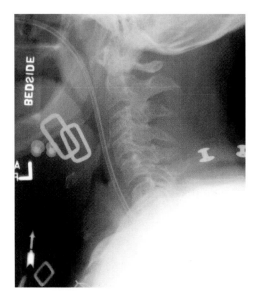

Fig. 4.56 Inadequate cervical spine film showing down to C6.

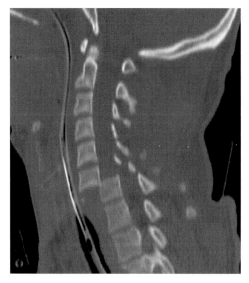

Fig. 4.57 CT sagittal reconstruction demonstrating fracture dislocation of the C6–C7.

The fracture is stable. If the patient is neurologically intact, further imaging with flexion extension views or CT scans of the affected level to rule out other occult fractures that might have been missed on plain film radiography is recommended. A rigid collar may be used as needed for pain.

The radiographic features on the lateral view reveal avulsion type fracture involving the spinous process and on the AP view a ghost sign is seen referring to a double spinous process of C6 and C7 (Fig. 4.55) resulting from usually caudal displacement of the fractured spinous process [2, 5, 6].

Complete radiographic assessment

The need to adequately image the cervical spine from C1 to C7–T1 cannot be overemphasised. The examples above (Figs 4.56 and 4.57) demonstrate the pitfalls of incomplete examination of the cervical spine. If the complete cervical spine cannot be visualised on plain films, then cross-sectional imaging is mandatory.

References

1. H.K. Lyerly, J.W. Gaynor. The Handbook of Surgical Intensive Care, 3rd edition, 1992.
2. John H. Harris Jr., Stuart E. Mirvis. The Radiology of the Acute Cervical Spine Trauma, 3rd edition, 1996.
3. R.K. MacDonald, M.L. Schwartz, D. Mirich, P.W. Sharkey, W.R. Nelson. Diagnosis of cervical spine injury in motor vehicle crash victims: how many X-rays are enough? J Trauma 1990; 30: 392–397.
4. Emergency and Trauma Radiology, 2000. Categorical Course Syllabus, American Roentgen Ray Society Meeting.
5. Adam Greenspan. Orthopedic Radiology. A Practical Approach, 3rd edition, 2000. Lippincott Williams and Wilkins, Philadelphia.
6. Mark S. Greenberg. Handbook of Neurosurgery, 5th edition, 2001.
7. R.H. Daffner. Thoracic and lumbar vertebral trauma. Orthopaedic Clinics of North America 1990; 21(3): 462–482.
8. P. Ford, J. Nolan. Cervical Spine Injury and Airway Management. Current Opinion in Anaesthesiology 2002; 15: 193–201.
9. S.B. Gay, R.J. Woodcock Jr. Radiology Recall, 2000.
10. N. Müller, Fraser, Colman, Pare. Radiologic Diagnosis of Disease of the Chest, 2001.

4

5

CT Head

Principles of CT image formation

How does CT work?

CT was discovered in 1972 by G.N. Hounsfield and since then its use has steadily grown so that now it is the workhorse of medical imaging. The original scanners took several minutes to take a single slice of the head but now the whole body can be scanned in 1–2 minutes. The scope of CT has increased from initially just head scans to current applications in all body systems.

A CT machine is comprised of the gantry, the table where the patient lies and the computer for operating the scanner and viewing images. The gantry is the large square giant donut with a patient aperture into which the patient is fed upon the table. The gantry is composed of a generator, X-ray tube, collimator and detectors. The gantry can be tilted to various degrees of angulation relative to a true perpendicular or axial slice. The X-ray tube circles the patient and produces a fan-shaped X-ray beam, the width of which is determined by collimators. The beam travels through the patient and is absorbed by a ring of detectors on the far side. The intensity of the X-rays reaching the detectors is recorded (an electrical current is generated that is proportional to the X-rays impinging on the detectors) and this depends on the absorbtion characteristics of the tissues through which the beam has passed. The X-ray beam is rotating around the patient so that each tiny block of tissue is exposed from multiple different directions. Using a sophisticated mathematical process called Fourier analysis, it is possible to allocate each tiny block of tissue a density value and exact position within the body. CT, although much more sophisticated than plain film radiography, relies on the same basic principle of dense structures blocking X-ray transmission. Each point on a CT image represents a volume of tissue or voxel. The units of relative density on CT are named after its inventor Hounsfield – Hounsfield units (HU). By definition, water has a density of 0 HU. An HU is a measure of linear attenuation coefficient compared to water. Further examples are listed below:

- bone: 400 HU,
- soft tissues: 80 HU,
- water: 0 HU,
- fat: −40.

A pixel is a two-dimensional representation of a three-dimensional block of tissue or voxel. Each pixel in the CT image is allocated a shade of grey depending on its density.

CT windows are a method of optimally displaying the shades of grey in a CT image. Windows have a level (the central HU valve) and a width, the range of CT valves displayed. In abdominal CT, the level may be 35 with a width of 400 – so that the CT demonstrates structures from −165 to +235 HU.

A narrow window like this is used when structures have similar densities in order to 'spread out' subtle changes in density. In the example above, values of greater than 235 would be shown as white and below -165 as black. Different CT windows are used to view different anatomical areas scanned, e.g. brain, posterior fossa, mediastinum, lung, liver, abdomen and bone all have different windows for image display.

What is spiral or helical CT?

The most significant advance in CT over the past few years has been the development of spiral CT. Conventional CT produces a data set for each individual slice scanned. The table moves to a location and the tube rotates to acquire data and the process is repeated for the next slice/position. There are cables in the gantry which means that between slices the tube has to reposition. Conventional machines are *start stop* scanners. Spiral CT continuously scans the patient as the table feeds through the gantry. X-ray exposure, table movement and data acquisition occur simultaneously. This produces a volume set of data of the entire region scanned. This is possible due to slip ring contacts (no constricting cables need to be unwound between slices). It is much quicker, and reduces problems from patient breathing – misregistration of images (on a conventional scanner a lesion may not appear on the scan if a patient takes a slightly different breath on two subsequent slices). The data set acquired is then reconstructed to represent axial slices. Images are easily reconstructed into different planes.

What is multi-slice CT?

With multi-slice CT, a single gantry rotation will capture multiple images, e.g. with quadslice CT, each gantry rotation captures four slices of data. The great advantage of multi-slice CT is its speed and its ability to cover large anatomical areas with thin collimation. There is no associated reduction in image quality. There are numerous applications including global trauma assessment (head, cervical spine, chest, abdomen and pelvis), vascular imaging, pulmonary embolism, virtual colonoscopy, lung cancer screening and cardiac imaging. One of the advantages of multi-detector CT is the ability to image organs in various phases of intravenous contrast enhancement – for instance, the pancreas can be scanned in arterial, parenchymal and portal venous phases with a single contrast injection.

Intravenous contrast medium

Intravenous contrast used in CT is an iodine-based contrast similar to that used for IVPs and numerous other radiological procedures. The iodine in the contrast causes X-ray absorption so that vascular structures and organs taking up the contrast medium appear more dense during the examination. This improves the contrast resolution between vascular and non-vascular structures. Contraindications to intravenous contrast include known contrast allergy, renal impairment and diabetic patients taking Metformin.

The contrast is administered via an intravenous cannula and the timing of administration is carefully controlled to coordinate with the timing of the CT scan. Various phases of contrast enhancement occur as the bolus of contrast passes from the arterial system into the veins and is finally excreted in the kidneys. The timing of the scan is dependent on the organ of interest and arterial phase, parenchymal, venous or delayed imaging (for instance, to show contrast in the ureters or bladder) can all be performed.

CT protocols

CT protocols are becoming more complex with the use of fast multi-slice scanners. Protocols are designed to optimally image a particular organ or body system. Other ways of optimising a scan include:

- patient positioning (prone or supine);
- breath holding;
- gantry tilt;
- varying CT slice thickness;
- oral contrast (either positive contrast or water contrast);
- rectal or bladder contrast;
- intravenous contrast;
- timing of the scan with respect to the intravenous contrast bolus;
- use of additional drugs, e.g. Buscopan to arrest bowel movement.

5

Principles of interpreting CT

CT head

The assessment of CT of the head depends on a good knowledge of normal brain anatomy. The left and right sides of the brain are basically symmetrical and the identification of asymmetry is invaluable in diagnosing pathology. The nature or composition of the tissues can be determined by looking at its density or Hounsfield value. There are broadly speaking only four categories of density. These are bone or calcification which is very dense and bright white, soft tissue density which is a variety of shades of grey, fat density which is dark grey and air which is black. By applying these principles, it is possible to determine the composition of a tissue seen on any CT scan, and a head CT scan in particular. Look at the different types of tissue in the normal anatomy sections – Question 1. The lateral ventricles and cerebral cisterns contain CSF which is water density, i.e. grey. Scalp fat is dark grey. All the bony structures and any calcification (for instance, in the choroid plexus) is bright white.

A CT scan takes axial slices through the head and by convention the anatomical right side is displayed to the right side of the page. It is like looking up at an axial section of the body from below. This should be obvious from the labelling of the scan.

CT head scans may be presented on either bony windows or brain windows. The reason for this is to optimise the appearance of the structures being investigated. Digital imaging has difficulty in displaying the full range of densities; so if a skull fracture is likely, then the images must be looked at on bone windows; but if the problem is intracerebral, then brain windows are necessary.

The majority of CT head scans performed for trauma are plain or without any intravenous contrast enhancement. It can be important to know whether a CT head scan was performed with or without contrast media. Often, the film will be labelled contrast or C. Contrast can be seen in the vessels or venous sinuses. Some lesions are dense, i.e. white without contrast enhancement and these can potentially be confused with avidly enhancing tumours, if it is not known whether contrast has been given.

Acute blood is dense or white on CT head scans, so it is possible to date a haematoma on the basis of its density. As the haematoma matures, the density gradually reduces (see Question 3). When fully mature, it can have almost the same density as CSF. The following cases and subsequent explanations demonstrate normal anatomy and the most commonly encountered pathologies seen in CT head examination. The pathologies are those most likely to be encountered in anaesthetic practice.

5

Case illustrations

Question 1

■ What are the normal anatomical structures labelled (Figs 5.1–5.4)?

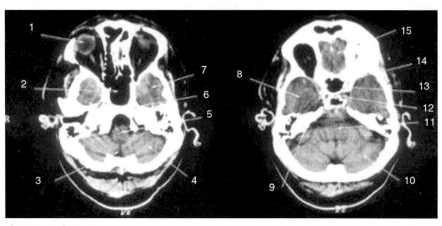

Fig. 5.1 Quiz case.

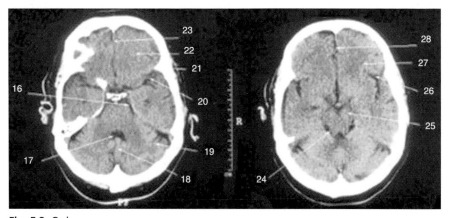

Fig. 5.2 Quiz case.

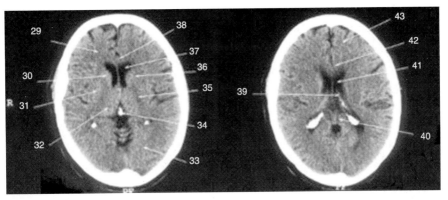

Fig. 5.3 Quiz case.

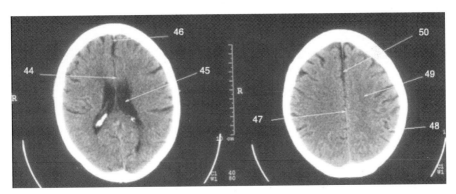

Fig. 5.4 Quiz case.

Answer

Normal anatomy

1. Right eye

2. Sphenoid sinus

3. Venous sinus

4. Left cerebellar hemisphere

5. Brain stem

6. Clivus

7. Left temporal lobe

8. Right temporal lobe

9. Sphenoid bone

10. Left cerebellar hemisphere

221

11. Brain stem

12. Pituitary fossa

13. Anterior clinoid process

14. Middle fossa

15. Olfactory lobes of frontal lobe

16. Ambient cistern

17. Fourth ventricle

18. Cerebellar vermis

19. Left cerebellar hemisphere

20. Sylvian fissure

21. Middle fossa

22. Left frontal lobe

23. Interhemispheric fissure

24. Quadrigeminal plate cistern

25. Cerebral peduncle

26. Sylvian fissure

27. White matter of left frontal lobe

28. Interhemispheric fissure

29. White matter of right frontal lobe

30. Head of caudate nucleus

31. Lentiform nucleus

32. Thalamus

33. Occipital lobe

34. Calcified pineal gland

35. Posterior limb of internal capsule

36. Anterior limb of internal capsule

37. Frontal horn of lateral ventricle

38. Corpus callosum

39. Choroid plexus

40. Corpus callosum

41. Body of lateral ventricle

42. Corpus callosum

43. Frontal lobe

44. Corpus callosum

45. Lateral ventricle

46. Interhemispheric fissure

47. Falcx

48. Sulcus

49. White matter

50. Interhemispheric fissure

Note the difference between the normal anatomy images above in a 40-year-old patient and the appearance in Fig. 5.5 which come from an 84-year-old patient. The brain volume is reduced with more prominent ventricles, cisterns and CSF spaces – there is cerebral atrophy.

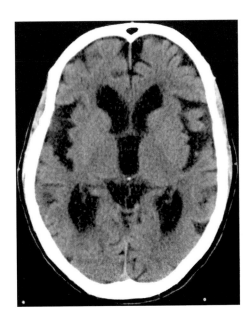

Fig. 5.5 This is the brain of an 84-year-old patient. The CSF spaces, ventricles and cisterns are more prominent than a younger patient and represent loss of brain volume or atrophy.

Question 2

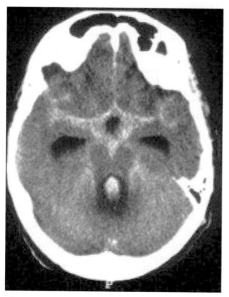

54-year-old female.
Sudden headache.
Reduced conscious level.

- What is the diagnosis (Fig. 5.6)?

- What is the initial anaesthetic management?

- What are the common causes?

- What further investigations are necessary?

- What are the complications?

Fig. 5.6 Quiz case.

Answer

Subarachnoid haemorrhage

There is blood in the sulci, the sylvian fissures bilaterally, in the basal cisterns and fourth ventricle. The temporal horns of the lateral ventricles are dilated due to hydrocephalus. This is likely to be due to obstruction of the aqueduct from haematoma.

The initial anaesthetic management depends on the patient's conscious level. All patients presenting with a reduced conscious level should be given high flow oxygen and an assessment made up of

- **A**irway,

- **B**reathing,

- **C**irculation,

- **D**ysfunction.

IV access should be maintained and monitoring attached. Any abnormalities in ABC should be treated immediately before moving on to the next phase of assessment. If the patient is comatose (Glasgow Coma Score (GCS) less than or equal to 8), they should be intubated and ventilated. A rapid sequence induction with cricoid pressure should be used to prevent aspiration. Intravenous anaesthetic agents and short-acting opioids should be used to prevent any further rise in intracranial pressure. The patient should be ventilated to normocapnoea and muscle relaxants and further anaesthetic drugs given to prevent coughing on the endotracheal tube. The patient should be accompanied by the anaesthetist to the CT scanner. A patient with a GCS of greater than 8 may need intubation for CT, if they are restless and uncooperative or if their airway is in anyway compromised. A patient with neurological injury should never be sedated for CT scan.

The initial anaesthetic management aims to keep the patient well oxygenated and normocapnic to prevent secondary brain injury. Blood pressure should be kept at a level to maintain cerebral perfusion pressure (CPP = MAP − [ICP + CVP]).

After the CT scan, the patient should be kept intubated and ventilated, and returned to an intensive therapy area while the case is discussed with the local neurosurgeons. The use of mannitol to decrease ICP and nimodipine for vasospasm should be discussed with them. If the regional neurosurgical unit is at another hospital, the patient should be transferred, intubated and ventilated by an experienced anaesthetist according to current guidelines [1].

Comment

Causes
- Berry aneurysm – 75%.

- AV malformation – 10%.

- Hypertension.

- Blunt trauma (see Fig. 5.7).

- No cause found.

Further investigations
An angiogram should be performed to identify any underlying cause. (see Fig. 5.8) cerebral angiogram.

Complications
1. Obstructive hydrocephalus from haematoma in the aqueduct.

2. Communicating hydrocephalus from failure of absorbtion by the arachnoid villi.

3. Vasospasm at 1 week producing brain infarction in associated territory.

4. Rebleeding at 2 weeks.

   Common sites for aneurysm formation is at the points of bifurcation:

- anterior communicating artery 30%,

- posterior communicating artery 30%,

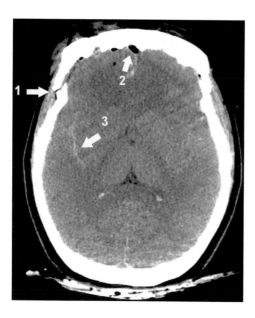

Fig. 5.7 Severe blunt head trauma: 1. skull fracture, 2. air within the skull vault, 3. traumatic subarachnoid blood.

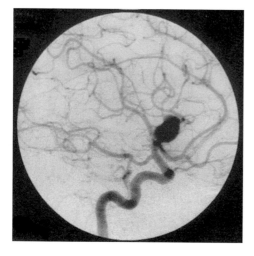

Fig. 5.8 This middle cerebral artery arteriogram shows a berry aneurysm at a point of bifurcation. The patient was being investigated for subarachnoid haemorrhage.

■ middle cerebral 25%,

■ terminal Internal carotid 12%.

Subarachnoid blood, when subtle, can be missed and a careful search should be made up of the sulci comparing right with the left side for differences in density. Further signs may be blood in the cisterns or layering in the lateral ventricles. If there is a high index of suspicion, a lumbar puncture looking for xanthochromia should be performed.

Question 3

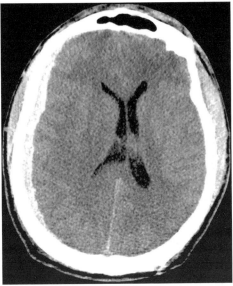

56-year-old male.
Alcoholic patient who has recently fallen.

Report the CT (Fig. 5.9).

■ How old is the abnormality?

■ What is the further management?

Fig. 5.9 Quiz case.

Answer

Acute subdural haematoma
There is a large high-density crescentic extra-axial collection around the right cerebral hemispheres with a concave inner margin and a convex outer margin. The collection traverses the skull sutures and is causing some mass effect with displacement of the midline to the left side.

The appearances are of an acute subdural collection. The high-density nature of the collection indicates that it is of recent onset, i.e. less than 1-week old.

Further management
Referral to a neurosurgical centre is indicated for consideration for drainage.

Comment
The subdural space lies superficial to the arachnoid, but deep to the dura and is not limited by sutures. The subdural space is limited by the interhemispheric fissure and the tentorium and subdural blood may be seen tracking along these structures. Subdural blood does not cross the midline. Extra-axial blood which is seen to cross a suture is likely to be subdural rather than extradural. Bleeding occurs when the bridging veins connecting the cerebral cortex and the dural sinuses are torn, e.g. trauma or deceleration injury. This happens when there is differential movement between the brain and the skull. Infants and the elderly are at greater risk

due to relatively large subarachnoid spaces (cerebral artophy in the elderly and alcoholics).

Subdural blood changes density with time allowing a collection to be dated:

- hyperdense: up to 1 week;

- isodense: 1–2 weeks (see Fig. 5.10);

- hypodense: 3–4 weeks, i.e. chronic subdural (Fig. 5.11).

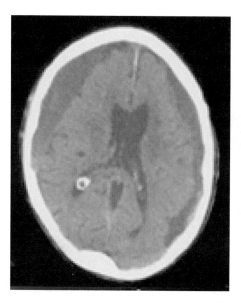

Fig. 5.10 Bilateral subacute subdural collections. From the density of these the age can be estimated at between 1 and 3 weeks of age. These can appear isodense to brain when they may be more difficult to identify especially when bilateral. If the sulci cannot be followed out to the brain surface subdural collections must be considered – widening the window can help.

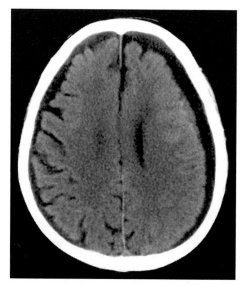

Fig. 5.11 Bilateral chronic subdural collections. These are of low-density (dark grey) dating them at 3–4 weeks or older.

It is reasonably easy to miss isodense subdural collections (subacute) check for

■ sulci reach the brain surface,

■ ipsilateral ventricular compression,

■ use a wide window width 400 and window level 40.

A membrane can form around chronic subdural collections (sometimes visible). Vessel fragility may cause rebleeding (see Fig. 5.12). In this situation, blood of different densities is frequently present (Fig. 5.13).

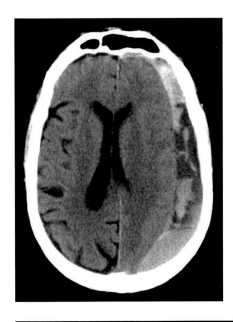

Fig. 5.12 Acute on chronic subdural. Rebleeding can occur after the initial acute event. Note, the vascular 'membrane' which is often the site of rebleeding.

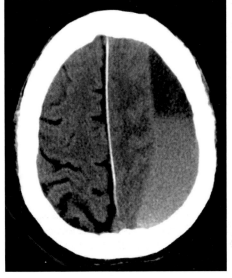

Fig. 5.13 Acute on chronic subdural. If blood has had time to mature before rebleeding occurs both acute blood (high density – white) and mature blood (low density – dark grey) are seen together. In this case the blood is seen layering out.

Question 4

Male aged 36.
Anaesthetic support has been requested for this patient who presented with a rapidly deteriorating conscious level following a head injury.

■ What are the key points in the anaesthetic management?

■ Report the CT (Fig. 5.14).

■ What is the pathogenesis?

■ What is the management?

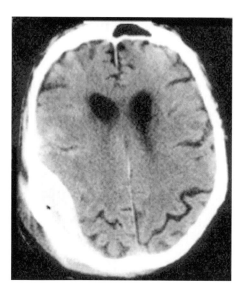

Fig. 5.14 Quiz case.

Answer

The patient should be managed as described in Question 2. In this case, the patient has had a head injury and so they must be considered to have a cervical spine injury until proven otherwise. During intubation inline cervical stabilisation must be performed and the hard collar, sandbags and tapes replaced after intubation. Ensure also that there are no other life-threatening traumatic injuries to the patient and that they are haemodynamically stable before going to the CT scan.

Extradural haematoma

There is a lens-shaped/biconcave high-density extra-axial collection in the right parietal region. Mass effect is minimal. This contains a small amount of air. The appearances are of an extradural haematoma. Laceration of the meningeal artery or vein from a skull fracture is the normal pathogenesis and the most common site is a temperoparietal location.

This is a neurosurgical emergency requiring urgent evacuation.

Comment

Up to 90% of extradural haematomas are associated with skull fracture. Contusion and subdural haematoma may also be associated. The mechanism of injury is usually laceration of the meningeal artery or vein. The often quoted text book history of concussion followed by a lucent interval only occurs in about a third of patients. More common is somnolence 24 hours or more following the head injury. An extradural haematoma particularly with mass effect is a neurosurgical emergency. Clues for diagnosis on CT are

- biconcave/lens shape,

- do not cross sutures,

- generally hyperdense to brain.

5

Question 5

72-year-old female.
Past history of poorly controlled hypertension.
Collapsed at home (Fig. 5.15).

- What is the diagnosis?

- What are the common causes?

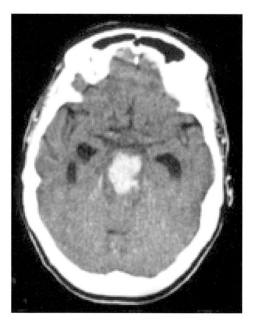

Fig. 5.15 Quiz case.

Answer

Intracerebral haematoma
There is a brain stem intracerebral haematoma causing hydrocephalus from ventricular obstruction at the level of the IV ventricle and aqueduct.

Common causes
- Hypertension
  - external capsule basal ganglia
  - pons
  - thalamus (see Fig. 5.16)
  - cerebellum

- Trauma

- Aneurysm

- Arteriovenous malformation

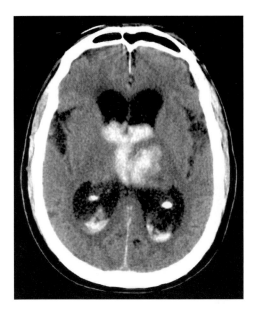

Fig. 5.16 Thalamic haemorrhage.

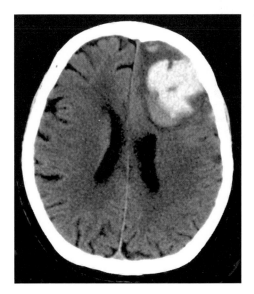

Fig. 5.17 Frontal haemorrhage. The patient was anticoagulated with warfarin.

■ Anticoagulation (see Fig. 5.17)

■ Haemorrhagic infarction (see Fig. 5.18).

Comment

The acute haematoma is normally rounded homogeneous and hyperdense. With clot retraction, a surrounding rim of low-density oedema appears. A non-contrast-enhanced CT scan is always performed, if intracerebral

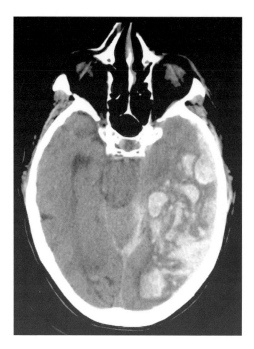

Fig. 5.18 Haemorrhagic infarct in the left middle cerebral artery territory. Note how the acute blood is limited to the middle cerebral artery territory.

haemorrhage is suspected. Otherwise it is not possible to distinguish acute blood from avid contrast enhancement (e.g. an avidly enhancing tumour).

Mass effect is often negligible and less than a tumour of a similar size. The haematoma can rupture into the ventriclular system and then cause hydrocephalus. Over a period of 1–2 weeks, the haematoma decreases in density starting in the periphery and working centrally. At this stage, contrast enhancement occurs peripherally due to formation of hypervascular granulation tissue.

Intracerebral haemorrhage is less common than infarction and a history of hypertension must be sought. Spontaneous rupture of the lenticulostriate arteries are frequently the cause and this explains why the basal ganglia are a common site.

Question 6

71-year-old male.
Slurred speech and hemiparesis.

■ Report the CT (Fig. 5.19).

■ What features of the history and physical examination are important?

■ What investigations should be performed?

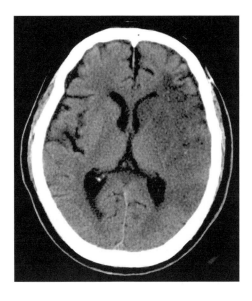

Fig. 5.19 Quiz case.

5

Answer

Infarction of the left middle cerebral artery territory
Assessment for risk factors for cerebrovascular disease are important in both the physical examination and the further investigations requested.

Physical examination
■ Hypertension

■ AF, heart murmurs, carotid bruits

■ Stigmata of raised cholesterol

Further investigations
■ ECG

■ Echocardiogram, carotid Doppler

■ Blood lipid profile

Comment

Cerebral infarction is rarely visible on CT prior to 12 hours, although newer scanners are improving resolution making earlier diagnosis possible. Early signs include:

- Hyperdense artery (from acute intraluminal thrombus) (see Fig. 5.20).

- Loss of grey–white interface.

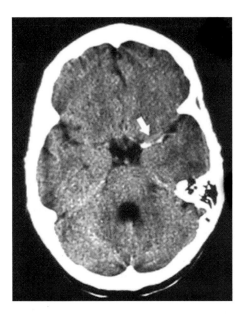

Fig. 5.20 Cerebral infarction is not readily identified before 12 hours duration. This scan demonstrates a hyperdense middle cerebral artery due to vessel thrombosis. A later scan confirmed infarction of the middle cerebral artery territory. A further early sign of infarction is loss of differentiation between grey and white matter.

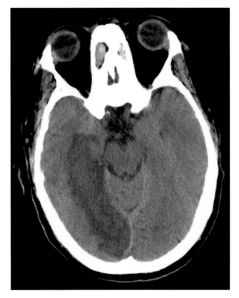

Fig. 5.21 Posterior cerebral artery territory infarction.

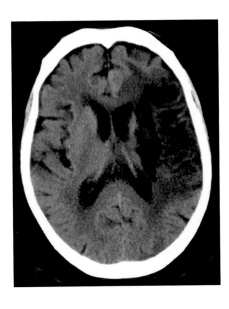

Fig. 5.22 Mature infarct in the territory of the left middle cerebral artery. Mature infarction is of lower density (darker black) than acute infarction.

The hallmark of ischaemia is a wedge-shaped low-density areas of affected brain which reaches the cortical surface. Middle cerebral artery infarction spares the thalamus. Mass effect is not uncommonly seen in the first week with sulcal effacement, ventricular and cisternal compression.

It is important to appreciate the territory supplied by the cerebral arteries as this enables confident diagnosis and helps distinguish infarction from space-occupying lesions. Space-occupying lesions cross arterial territories while infarction is limited by them. Infarction in the territory of the middle cerebral artery (hemiparesis) and the posterior cerebral artery (see Fig. 5.21) (producing homonymous hemianopia) are the more commonly affected arteries. The anterior cerebral artery territory is rarely affected partly due to good collateral supply from the anterior communicating artery. On CT an area of mature infarction is of reduced density and appears darker than acute infarction (Fig. 5.22).

Question 7

58-year-old female.
Admitted following road traffic accident and minor head injury (Fig. 5.23).
Normal physical examination.
No fracture could be seen on the film and the patient was discharged from accident and emergency.

■ What is the radiological abnormality on the plain film of the skull?

■ Suggest two possible differential diagnoses.

■ What radiological investigation would you want to request next?

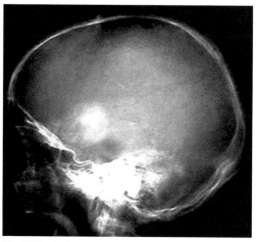

Fig. 5.23 Quiz case.

Answer

Meningioma

No skull fracture is present. There is a 3 cm diameter oval opacity of calcific density projected over the skull vault. Possibilities would include a calcified meningioma or possibly a giant calcified aneurysm. A frontal skull X-ray should be reviewed to confirm that the lesion is within the skull vault. A CT scan of the brain would be a suitable next request (see Fig. 5.24).

The CT scan demonstrates a densely calcified lesion arising from the middle cranial fossa which is extra-axial (outside of the brain). These are features characteristic of a calcified meningioma.

One of the great advantages of MRI scanning is its multiplanar capability and coronal imaging clearly confirms the extra-axial nature of the lesion (see Fig. 5.25).

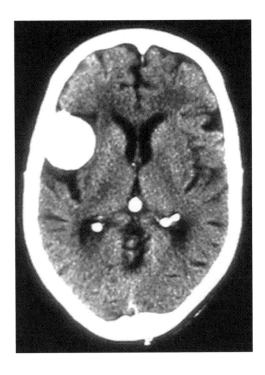

Fig. 5.24 CT of a densely calcified meningioma.

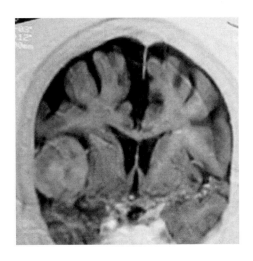

Fig. 5.25 MRI of meningioma. The extra-axial nature of the meningioma is clearly seen on this coronal MRI scan. The brain can be seen displaced, but separate from the tumour.

Comment

Meningioma is the most common extra-axial intracranial tumour often found incidentally. Presentation is usually in middle age unless associated with neurofibromatosis type 2 when it occurs in childhood and can be multiple. Meningiomas occur at sites where arachnoid villi are in proximity to the dura such as the venous sinuses.

239

Locations:

- cerebral hemispheres;

- parasagittal;

- middle fossa and sphenoid bone;

- posterior fossa, cerebellopontine angle, spinal.

Cerebellopontine angle meningiomas may mimic acoustic neuromas. Hyperostosis with skull vault thickening and sclerosis may be present on plain films. CT-imaging features are of a well-circumscribed, slow-growing dense lesion, which may calcify. Enhancement is avid and homogeneous. The prognosis is generally better compared with gliomas and metastatic lesions which are both more common.

5

Question 8

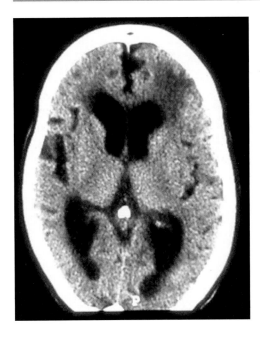

55-year-old female.
History – known breast carcinoma.
Recent headaches.
Possible cerebral metastases (Fig. 5.26).

- What is the abnormality?

- What further test is necessary?

Fig. 5.26 Quiz case.

Answer

Cerebral metastasis

There is an area of low density in the region of the left frontal lobe. This is rather asymmetric when compared with the right side.

Intravenous contrast enhancement should be given in view of the history of breast carcinoma.

Following IV contrast (Fig. 5.27) there is a 1 cm diameter area of avid contrast enhancement. This is a cerebral metastasis and the low density surrounding it is white matter oedema.

Situations requiring IV contrast include:

- suspected malignancy primary or secondary,

- inflammatory conditions such as abscess,

- vascular lesions such as arteriovenous malformations,

- venous sinus thrombosis (to *demonstrate failure in opacification?* and filling defects in the sinus).

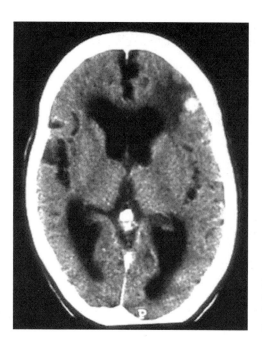

Fig. 5.27 Breast metastasis enhancing following IV contrast. The surrounding low density is oedema.

Question 9

49-year-old male.
History – bizarre behaviour for several weeks more rapid deterioration over past few days.

- Describe the abnormal radiological signs (Figs 5.28 and 5.29).

- What is the differential diagnosis?

- What urgent management should be considered?

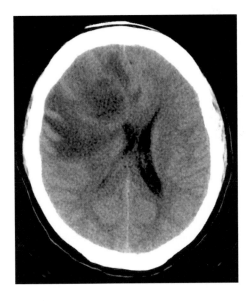

Fig. 5.28 Quiz case.

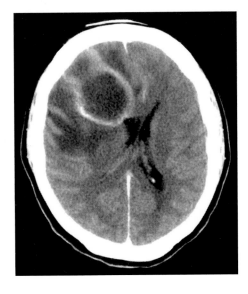

Fig. 5.29 Quiz case.

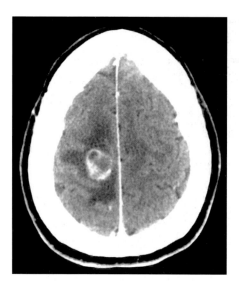

Fig. 5.30 Ring-enhancing lesion post-contrast. This is a further example of a malignant glioma. The differential for this lesion includes an abscess and clinical correlation is necessary (clinical history, temperature, inflammatory markers – CRP, leucocyte count). Abscesses are typically thin walled with surrounding oedema.

Answer

Malignant brain glioma

There is a ring enhancing lesion in the right frontal lobe which is surrounded by extensive oedema. The abnormality has marked mass effect with deviation of the midline to the left side, effacement of the frontal horn of the right lateral ventricle and basal cisterns is present.

The differential diagnosis for intracerebral ring enhancing lesions includes:

■ primary brain tumour (glioblastoma multiforme) (see Fig. 5.30),

■ metastases (see Fig. 5.31),

■ cerebral lymphoma,

■ abscess (pyogenic or fungal),

■ resolving haematoma (which is surrounded by granulation tissue).

Given the history of gradual deterioration pyogenic abscess is unlikely. Corticosteroids to reduce the oedema can improve symptoms in the short term. This lesion was biopsied and was found to be a glioblastoma multiforme.

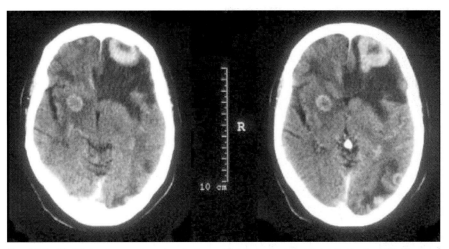

Fig. 5.31 Multiple ring-enhancing lesions. This appearance is typical of multiple cerebral metastases. The presence of a primary lesion helps with the diagnosis.

Comment

Neurosurgical assessment and sampling of the lesion to exclude pyogenic abscess should be considered if there are signs of sepsis or an obvious source of infection. If the clinical picture is that of sepsis, then possible sources would include frontal sinusitis, mastoiditis or blood-borne infection from endocarditis. The latter tends to give rise to multiple abscesses. The possibility of AIDS or altered immunity should be kept in mind with multiple abscesses as cerebral toxoplasmosis appears very similar to pyogenic abscess.

Question 10

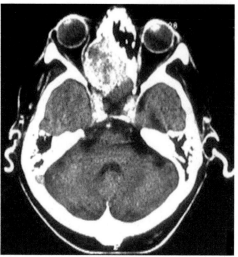

64-year-old male.
Recurrent nose bleeds.
Renal carcinoma removed
18 months ago.

- What is the abnormality
  (Fig. 5.32)?

Fig. 5.32 Quiz case.

Answer

Metastasis

There is a soft tissue density mass measuring 4 cm × 2.5 cm in diameter
occupying the paranasal air sinuses particularly on the right side. This is
destroying bone and eroding into the medial wall of the right orbit.
A malignant process is likely.

Comment

The case above was a metastatic deposit from renal cell carcinoma.
It illustrates the need to interrogate the whole film and in particular to
look at certain sites where disease is commonly missed. These review areas
must be checked before the film is reported.

Review areas:

- skull base (for malignant disease);

- pituitary fossa (tumours);

- sinuses;

- temporal lobes (low density in herpes simplex encephalitis);

- sulci (for isodense subdural or subarachnoid blood);

- 'top slice' (parafalcine meningioma);

- cisterns (blood, e.g. SAH);

- bone windows for fractures or metastatic disease in the skull vault.

Question 11

48-year-old female.
Headaches.

■ Suggest a differential diagnosis for this abnormality (Fig. 5.33).

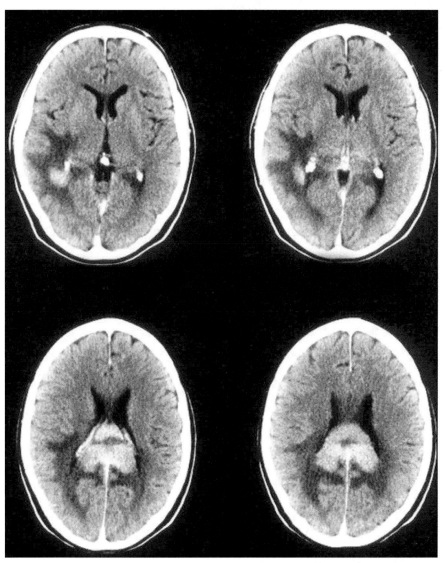

Fig. 5.33 Quiz case.

Answer

- Butterfly glioma

- Metastasis

- Cerebral lymphoma

Comment

Glioma is the generic term used to encompass glial cell tumours growing along white matter tracts.

Different types exist including:

- glioblastoma multiforme,

- astrocytoma,

- ependymoma,

- oligodendroglioma.

Characterisation can be difficult on the basis of imaging.

Glioblastoma multiforme which accounts for roughly half of brain tumours typically has a multilobulated appearance. They occur in the hemispheres or posterior fossa but when in the splenium of the corpus callosum these are described as butterfly gliomas due to the appearance and spread across the midline.

5

Question 12

27-year-old male.
Head injury following high alcohol consumption.
Reduced conscious level.

You are called to the accident and emergency department to help manage this patient:

■ How would you prevent secondary brain injury?

■ What parameters need careful monitoring?

■ What is the abnormality on CT (Fig. 5.34)?

■ What is the short-term management?

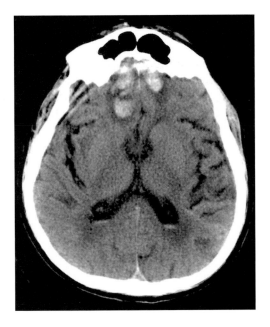

Fig. 5.34 Quiz case.

Answer

Head injury accounts for approximately a third of all trauma deaths and is the leading cause of death and disability in young adults.

Secondary brain injury occurs after the initial insult and is the result of cerebral hypoxia and ischaemia. Assess and act on abnormalities found to prevent further insult to the vulnerable brain.

■ **A**irway (with cervical spine control)
- Prevent hypoxia aim for a clear unobstructed airway and $SpO_2 > 95\%$.
- If there is airway compromise intubate with a rapid sequence induction, cricoid pressure and inline cervical spine stabilisation. Pass an orogastric tube.

- **B**reathing
  - Ventilate if the patient is intubated for airway protection or for ventilatory failure.
  - Aim for $PaCO_2$ of 4.0–4.5 kPa avoid hyper/hypocapnia.
- **C**irculation
  - Keep systolic BP > 120 mmHg (maintain CPP > 70 mmHg).
  - Two large IV cannula should be sited.
- **D**ysfunction
  - Assess neurological state using GCS (Table 5.1) and AVPU.
  - Prevent further neurological injury treat seizures and hyperglycaemia.
  - Prevent hyperthermia.
  - Maintain ICP <20–25 mmHg (if monitoring available).
  - Evidence of raised ICP – pupillary dilatation, motor posturing, progressive neurological deficit, consider mannitol (0.25–0.5 g/kg). Ensure adequate sedation.
  - Nurse 30° head up, do not obstruct venous return.
- **E**xternal examination
  - Exclude extracranial injuries.

Table 5.1 **The GCS is scored between 3 and 15 (maximum score 15, minimum 3). It is composed of three parameters**

Best eye response (4)	
Spontaneous eye opening	4
Eye opening to speech	3
Eye opening to pain	2
No eye opening	1
Best motor response (6)	
Obeys commands	6
Localises to pain	5
Withdraws from pain	4
Abnormal flexion to pain	3
Extension to pain (decerebrate)	2
No movement	1
Verbal response (5)	
Orientated (able to give name and age)	5
Confused (still answers questions)	4
Inappropriate words	3
Incomprehensible sounds (grunts, no actual words)	2
None	1

It is helpful to breakdown the component score of the GCS, e.g. E4V3M4 = GCS 11. A coma score of 13 or higher correlates with mild brain injury, 9–12 with moderate brain injury and 8 or below with a severe brain injury.

5

Frontal lobe haematomas and cerebral contusion

A wide range of appearances are seen on CT head scans performed for severe head injury. A large proportion of trauma head scans follow road traffic accidents. Haemorrhage is frequently seen in more than one compartment (Fig. 5.35) demonstrates traumatic subarachnoid blood and subdural blood in the same patient. This patient sustained a severe injury and the follow-up scan (Fig. 5.36) demonstrates several pockets of air

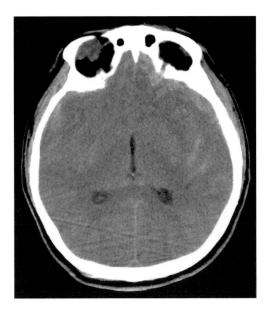

Fig. 5.35 CT head scan performed for blunt trauma following a motor vehicle accident. Acute subdural blood seen peripherally and acute traumatic subarachnoid blood is present interdigitating along the sulci.

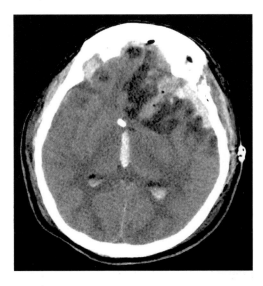

Fig. 5.36 This is a CT head scan 3 days following blunt head injury (same patient as Fig. 5.35). There is contusion and now quite extensive infarction, and both traumatic subarachnoid and subdural blood is still present.

within the brain and extensive low-density changes in keeping with infarction. Subdural blood is still present. Traumatic subarachnoid blood is a not infrequent finding in the setting of trauma and can be present in isolation as in Figs 5.37 and 5.38 where there is subarachnoid blood around the frontal lobes and in the basal cisterns as well as gross brain swelling. Note, how the brain is of reduced density and there is loss of

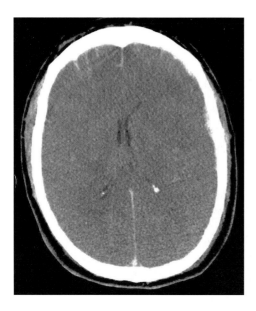

Fig. 5.37 Traumatic subarachnoid haemorrhage. This is best seen as 'fingers' of high density in the sulci peripherally. The brain is very swollen and oedematous with loss of distinct differentiation between grey and white matter. The brain is of reduced density.

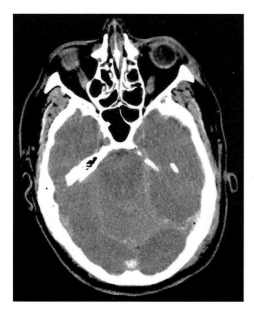

Fig. 5.38 Traumatic subarachnoid haemorrhage with blood in the basal cisterns.

differentiation between grey and white matter. It is important to view CT scans of the head performed for trauma on a number of different window settings. Skull fractures are much more apparent on bone windows (see Figs 5.39 and 5.40) than on the corresponding soft tissue windows. In the trauma setting it is important to search for air within or surrounding the brain as this is indicative of a skull fracture (Figs 5.41 and 5.42). More subtle appearances on CT can, nevertheless, be indicative of severe injury and are associated with considerable morbidity. Figures 5.43 and 5.44 demonstrate

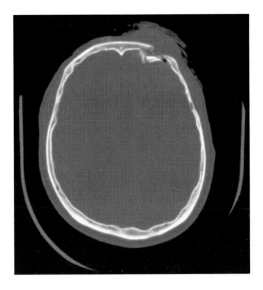

Fig. 5.39 CT head following motor cycle accident (no helmet). There is a depressed skull fracture with a small pocket of air within the cranium. The bony anatomy is most clearly visualised on bone windows.

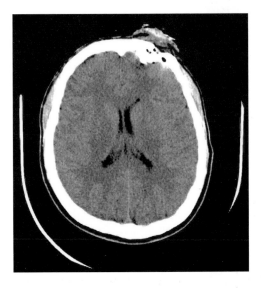

Fig. 5.40 CT head displayed on normal brain window (same scan as Fig. 5.39) to demonstrate the difference between brain and bone window. The brain window is clearly superior for demonstrating the brain contusion and haematoma.

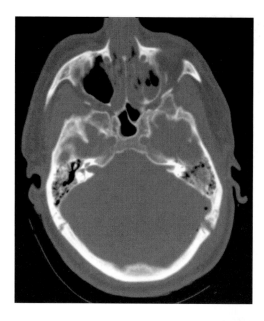

Fig. 5.41 Posterior fossa fracture with small amount of pneumocephalus displayed on bone window.

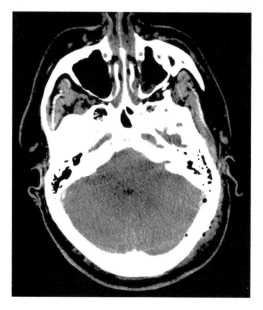

Fig. 5.42 Pneumocephalus and fracture displayed on brain window.

traumatic petechial haemorrhages seen in the brain stem and right frontal cortex of a patient involved in a high speed motor vehicle accident.

The extent of these shear injuries is often underestimated on CT and more widespread changes can frequently be demonstrated on MRI. These white matter shearing injuries occur in the setting of a diffuse impact injury with rotational forces. The cortex and deep structures move at different speeds resulting in shearing stress especially at grey–white matter junctions.

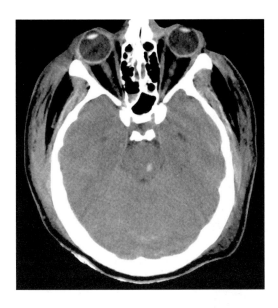

Fig. 5.43 White matter shearing injury. CT head scan following high speed motor vehicle accident. There is a tiny acute haematoma in the brain stem. CT is relatively poor at demonstrating tiny haemorrhagic lesions which are better seen on MRI.

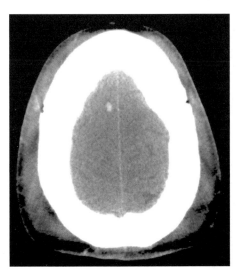

Fig. 5.44 Tiny haematoma in frontal lobe. MRI demonstrated multiple similar lesions.

Reference

1. Neuroanaesthesia Society of Great Britain and Ireland and the Association of Anaesthetists of Great Britain and Ireland. Recommendations for the Transfer of Patients with Acute Head Injuries to Neurosurgical Units, 1996.

6

Anaesthesia in the radiology department with particular reference to MRI and interventional radiology

Anaesthesia in the radiology department

Anaesthesia in the radiology department produces challenges for the anaesthetist which include:

1. equipment, which is not in current use elsewhere in the hospital;

2. inadequate monitoring devices;

3. piped medical gases may not be supplied;

4. radiology personnel may be unaware of anaesthetic problems;

5. bulky equipment may limit space around, and access to the patient;

6. the magnetic field and radiofrequency (RF) currents in magnetic resonance imaging (MRI) require special precautions;

7. lighting may be poor and the environment may be colder than an operating theatre;

8. recovery facilities may not be available.

The most important message from these is 'skilled anaesthetic assistance is essential'. The Association of Anaesthetists of Great Britain and Ireland (AAGBI) has made recommendations for the standards of monitoring during anaesthesia [1] which is essential reading for all anaesthetists. One section of this document states, 'The AAGBI regards it as essential that certain core standards of monitoring must be used whenever a patient is anaesthetised. These standards should be uniform irrespective of duration or *location* of anaesthesia.'

These recommendations also state, 'When there is a known potential hazard to the anaesthetist, for example during imaging procedures, facilities for remotely observing and monitoring the patient must be available.'

Guidelines also exist to ensure the safe management of sedated and anaesthetised patients in radiology [2, 3], although unfortunately these are often not adhered to in many departments. The current guidelines (1992) of the Royal College of Anaesthetists and the Royal College of Radiologists [2] suggest that a designated consultant anaesthetist should take responsibility for anaesthetic matters in the radiology department. Their responsibilities should include:

- ensuring adequate provision of resuscitation equipment and drugs,

- advising on the design of rooms where sedation and anaesthesia are to be administered,

- the provision of recovery areas,

- establishing guidelines for sedation in radiology,

- training radiologists in the management of sedated patients.

These guidelines are currently being updated in response to the increasing numbers of complex procedures carried out in radiology, and to the Joint College's document on sedation practices [3].

Hazards to anaesthetists

Radiation exposure to the anaesthetist working with investigative radiology procedures is not normally high. The real radiation risks occur during interventional procedures where 'screening' is frequently performed. However, adequate protective precautions should always be taken. The anaesthetist should distance themselves as far as possible from the radiation source during imaging. Pregnant anaesthetists should avoid involvement in radiological procedures.

Anaesthesia for diagnostic radiology

The anaesthetist is most commonly involved in the management of patients having computerised tomography (CT) or MRI investigations. The patients can be divided into elective and emergency categories.

Elective investigations require sedation or anaesthesia to render the small child, or rarely the uncooperative adult, immobile. Most diagnostic radiological procedures are not painful, but the patient must remain motionless during the examination. The newest CT systems can generate images very rapidly and MRI is getting faster; however, some of the more complex examinations in MRI may still take up to 20 minutes for one scan and up to 1 hour for the whole examination.

Emergency patients require the presence of an anaesthetist for their safe management and *they should not be moved from the resuscitation area until they are stable*. Movement around the hospital of recently admitted trauma, or seriously ill medical patients for investigation should be as rigorously planned as inter-hospital transfer. The sections on equipment, preparation for transfer, and monitoring of the Intensive Care Society Guidelines [4] for transport of the critically ill adult, can be equally applied to the in-hospital transfer of patients from Accident and Emergency or ICU to Radiology. Intubation for all emergency patients should be performed with a rapid sequence induction and cricoid pressure on a tipping trolley. Once the airway has been established, checked and secured the patient can then be transferred onto the X-ray table.

Anaesthesia or sedation?

There are many articles discussing the relative merits of anaesthesia or sedation for radiological investigations, and many different sedative and anaesthetic techniques have been used. Whichever option is chosen, all patients should be seen, fully assessed, and have had appropriate investigations performed. Patients may attend as day cases and day case management should be applied. When planning anaesthesia or

6

sedation for radiological procedures, the length of procedure, accessibility of the airway, underlying medical condition and the need for rapid recovery must be considered, and the most appropriate agents used.

Not all patients require general anaesthesia or sedation; infants may sleep through relatively long examinations, if the study is performed after a feed and they are well wrapped up to keep them warm. Play therapy has been effective in persuading children over the age of 4 years to undergo MRI without anaesthesia or sedation. Adults who suffer from severe anxiety or claustrophobia can be positioned prone in the magnet bore, reassured and if necessary counselled before anaesthesia or sedation is attempted.

Although many anaesthetists in UK choose anaesthesia to render small children immobile for radiological investigation, worldwide sedation is most commonly used. In children's hospitals, multidisciplinary sedation teams have demonstrated excellent success rates and safety records for sedation for radiological procedures. What appears to be important is not the use of a specific sedative or regimen, but the presence of an organised team dedicated exclusively to paediatric sedation, which deals with relatively large numbers of patients. Sedating children, however, particularly in non-specialist centres, can be difficult and unpredictable, the advantages of general anaesthesia are that it has a more rapid and controlled onset and immobility is guaranteed. Sick children may be better managed with general anaesthesia; certainly if there is any question of raised intracranial pressure, then sedation is inappropriate and potentially dangerous.

If anaesthesia is chosen, short-acting agents should be used. Investigative procedures are usually painless and therefore the use of potent long-acting opioids is inappropriate. Total intravenous anaesthesia may be ideal due to its rapid recovery characteristics and low incidence of induced nausea and vomiting. It is worth remembering when planning anaesthesia (or sedation) for MRI that infusion pumps will malfunction above a certain level of magnetic field strength (30 G). The airway should be secured in whatever way is suitable for that patient and for the procedure. It is generally inappropriate, even if it is possible, to hold the patient's airway during an X-ray procedure as the anaesthetist is then forced to remain close to the radiation source. The laryngeal mask offers the ideal alternative for the patient who does not need endotracheal intubation.

At the end of the procedure, the patient should be transferred to a recovery area and managed by trained recovery personnel. They should not be discharged to the ward until they have met standard post-anaesthetic care unit discharge criteria.

The anaesthetist working in the radiology department must balance the needs of the radiologist, and increasingly the surgical team, whilst maintaining adequate anaesthesia, patient homeostasis and minimising risks to the patient, staff and themselves.

MRI: principles of image formation

How is an MR image produced?

MRI uses a magnetic field rather than X-rays/ionising radiation to produce an image. To perform an MRI scan, the patient is placed in very strong magnetic field (superconducting magnet) of the MRI scanner. The hydrogen nuclei/protons within the body are subjected to bursts of radiofrequency (RF). The hydrogen nuclei in the body take up the RF energy, which is subsequently released again as they relax. This emitted energy is measured using an external RF coil. This signal can be localised to an exact location in the body and varies depending on the physical composition of the emitting body part. These signals are built up into MR images.

MRI depends on the interaction between several factors:

1. Hydrogen nuclei (single protons) within tissues, mostly within water molecules.

2. A strong and uniform external magnetic field (0.15–2 T).

3. Pulses of RF/radiowaves.

The hydrogen nuclei act like tiny spinning bar magnets (magnetic moments) and within the MRI scanner they align themselves parallel or anti-parallel to the external magnetic field. If radiowaves/RF of a critical frequency (the resonant or Lamor frequency) are generated, some of the nuclei absorb energy causing them to change their orientation relative to the external magnetic field. This causes rotation of the net magnetisation vector to rotate through a certain angle – flip angle, e.g. 90 degrees. The greater the strength and duration of the RF pulse, the greater the flip angle. At the same time, all of the nuclei begin to spin in phase with one another. When the RF is turned off, the nuclei start to relax towards their resting state. The magnetisation vector returns to its original orientation (T1 relaxation). Immediately following the RF pulse, the individual magnetic moments are rotating in phase. Simultaneously with T1 relaxation, there is dephasing of the spins (T2 relaxation). As relaxation occurs, the signal decays. Every tissue has its own T1 and T2 relaxation rates, which depend on the chemical and physical properties of that tissue. T2 relaxation or spin–spin relaxation is a much more rapid process. The small alternating magnetic field, perpendicular to the external field, induces an electrical current in receiver coils placed close to the patient. This current is amplified into an MRI signal.

In MRI, the field gradients are employed to make the MRI signal contain spatial information. The gradient field is superimposed on the main magnetic field for spatial encoding. There are three orthogonal gradient coils – in the transverse (X and Y) and longitudinal (Z) planes. This allows localisation of the signal which can then be translated onto the final image. It is the gradient coil which produces the loud banging during an MRI study. The strength of the signal from a given point in the patient

6

determines the shade of grey of the corresponding pixel on the image. High signal tissue appears white and low signal black, with a spectrum in between.

How is tissue contrast created?

A long train of radiowave pulses make up the imaging sequence.
The duration and timing of the pulses determine which tissue properties will be reflected in the final image, e.g. the T1 or T2 relaxation rates (T1- or T2-weighted image). Images may also be weighted for the proton density of tissues, which corresponds to their free-water content. Therefore, unlike CT, tissue contrast in MRI is variable, and an understanding of the sequence used is required in order to interpret images.

TE is the time to echo, or the time between applying the RF pulse and listening for the signal. TR is the time to repeat or the time between RF pulses. TR and TE are measured in milliseconds (ms).

By looking at the TR and TE (which is normally printed on the sheet of film), it is possible to decide whether the image has been T1 or T2 weighted:

- T1 weighted
  - short TR: 600 ms,
  - short TE: 20 ms.

- T2 weighted
  - long TR: 3000 ms,
  - long TE: 80 ms.

The alternative way of deciding whether a sequence is T1 or T2 weighted is by looking at the signal returned by certain types of tissue. For instance, water is low signal on T1- and high signal on T2-weighted images (see Fig. 6.1). By looking at the bladder or CSF spaces, it should be possible to decide what sort of image has been taken.

Useful signal intensities

- T1-weighted image
  - Fluid: low signal (black).
  - Fat: high signal (white).
  - Enhancement with IV gadolinium: high signal.
  - Blood methaemoglobin (subacute haemorrhage): high signal.
  - Melanin: high signal.

- T2-weighted image
  - Fluid: high signal.
  - Fat: high/intermediate signal.
  - Mature haemorrhage (haemosiderin): low signal.

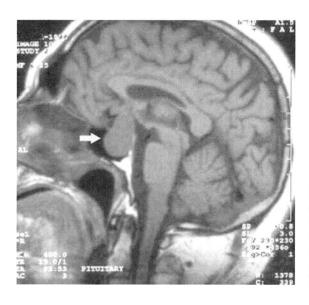

Fig. 6.1 T1-weighted sagittal MRI image through the brain. Note the CSF is dark grey, fat is white and brain is mid-grey. Note also the large pituitary tumour.

Some tissues show low signal (black) on all sequences:

- cortical bone,
- calcification,
- tendons/ligaments,
- menisci in the knee,
- gas.

The signal intensity from flowing blood is variable and depends on several factors including the sequence used, and the speed and direction of flow. On spin-echo (SE) images, flowing blood usually produces no signal (flow-void). Most pathological processes result in an increase in the water content of tissues, and they therefore tend to be most conspicuous, as areas of increased signal, on T2-weighted images.

Some commonly used MRI sequences

- Spin-echo (SE): the most widely used and versatile sequences. May be T1-, T2- or proton-density weighted.
- Turbo spin-echo (TSE) and gradient echo (GE): fast sequences.
- STIR: high signal from fat is suppressed, so that high signal pathology and fluid stand out.
- FLAIR: high signal from CSF is suppressed – good for detecting subtle brain lesions.

MR angiography (MRA)

May be used to study arteries or veins (MRV). Flowing blood produces a high signal, whilst all signal from the surrounding, static tissue is suppressed. MRA is non-invasive, does not involve radiation or potentially harmful contrast agents, and has an accuracy approaching conventional angiography in some diagnostic situations.

Contrast agents in MRI

Despite the excellent inherent tissue contrast in MR images, intravenous contrast medium is often given to highlight abnormal tissue. Chelates of the paramagnetic substance gadolinium are used – they shorten the relaxation times of nearby protons which results in high signal on T1-weighted images. Gadolinium has similar pharmacokinetics to the iodinated contrast media used in CT – it is distributed throughout the intra- and extravascular spaces, does not cross the intact blood–brain barrier, is hyperosmolar and excreted renally – caution is needed in patients with renal failure. The frequency of adverse reactions is around 2–5%, although most are mild (nausea, urticaria, etc.). Anaphylactoid reactions are rare, but have been reported.

MRI vs. CT

MRI and CT are not generally interchangeable examinations, the choice depends on the likely pathology and the body part in question. CT is superior to MRI in demonstrating calcified or ossified lesions (these show no signal on MRI). CT remains the imaging modality of choice for most chest, abdominal and pelvic pathology.

Advantages of MRI

1. No ionising radiation.

2. Superior soft tissue contrast.

3. Direct multiplanar capabilities (however, the newer helical CT scanners are able to reconstruct images in any plane from the data that is acquired axially).

Disadvantages of MRI

1. Longer imaging times (minutes vs. seconds) mean that images may be degraded by patient movement, breathing, bowel peristalsis and cardiac pulsation. The latter is reduced by the use of cardiac gating techniques, whereby data is only acquired during a certain short part of the cardiac cycle.

2. Most MR scanners are not patient friendly – they are very enclosed and noisy such that claustrophobic patients and children may not tolerate a scan. Combined with the relatively long scanning times means that children are more likely to require sedation or general anaesthetic.

6

3. All monitoring and resuscitation equipment to be used within the scanner must be MRI compatible.

4. Contraindications to MRI are not uncommon.

Safety issues in MRI
(see also MRI and anaesthesia section)

Contraindications to MRI
Absolute

- Cardiac pacemakers.

- Implanted cardiac defibrillators.

- Cochlear implants.

- Any other implanted device which is electrically/magnetically operated.

- Metallic ocular foreign bodies (X-ray orbits if any doubt).

- Cerebrovascular aneurysm clips and some other ferromagnetic implants.

Relative
Pregnancy – there is no evidence as yet that MRI has any harmful effects on the foetus, however data is limited. There is a theoretical risk of teratogenicity in the first trimester, and MRI should be particularly avoided at this time. However, a clinical decision has to be made as to whether the benefits of the examination outweigh any potential risk. Pregnant staff should be able to opt out of working in the MRI suite, if they wish.

MRI: anaesthetic monitoring

MRI produces additional challenges to the anaesthetist [5, 6], in addition to those described earlier, due to the effects of the magnetic field and RF currents used in MRI.
   The main problems are

- the high magnetic field with associated risks of ferromagnetic attraction,

- the narrow magnet bore in which the patient is completely enclosed,

- malfunction of monitoring equipment,

- degradation of the MR images by the presence of monitoring equipment.

The advent of low field 'open' MR systems reduces some of the anaesthetist's problems; the patient is visible, access to them is easier and the environment is less claustrophobic. However, the 'open' magnet operates at low field strength and is suitable only for certain types of investigation.

Magnetic field strength and ferromagnetic attraction

Magnetic field strength is measured in tesla (T). One tesla is equal to 10,000 G. The earth's magnetic field at the surface is in the order of 0.5–2.0 G. Clinical MRI systems in the UK operate between 0.05 and 2.0 T, that is 500–20,000 times the earth's surface magnetic field. The anaesthetist should know the extent of the magnetic field he or she is working in. A useful measure is the 5 G line, this is the field strength at which pacemakers will dysfunction, electrical equipment may start to malfunction and magnetic tape such as that on credit cards will be erased. Infusion pumps will malfunction at a field strength of 30 G. At a field strength of approximately 50 G the attractive force on ferromagnetic objects becomes significant, and an object such as oxygen cylinder can become a dangerous projectile accelerating into the magnet bore, 'the missile effect'!
The anaesthetist should consider the magnetic field to be permanently on.
It is very expensive to shut down the field and not without risk.
Never assume that in case of emergency the magnetic field can be turned off.

Patient and staff hazards

All MRI units operate certain patient and personnel exclusions because of the risks of ferromagnetic attraction. Everybody entering the unit should complete a screening questionnaire. Pacemakers, automatic defibrillators, infusion pumps and neurostimulators may malfunction at very low field strengths and patients with these devices should not be allowed anywhere near the magnetic field. Many implanted prosthetic devices are non-ferromagnetic. Objects of unknown ferrous content can be tested with a hand-held magnet. Some ferromagnetic items pose little threat to the patient as they are firmly anchored, such as joint prostheses. They will, however, cause artefacts when scanned with MR which can severely degrade the images. There are some items where any movement would be critical, such as intra-cerebral aneurysm clips or intra-ocular metallic fragments, and patients with these *in situ* must not be placed in the magnetic field unless their non-magnetic content is known unequivocally. The newer types of heart valves are not ferromagnetic and flow changes or heating do not seem to cause problems. There are extensive and frequently updated reviews of the magnetic susceptibilities of biomedical implants available. No patient should be taken near an MR system, if there is any query about the safety of any prosthetic device, implant or surgical clip as disasters have occurred. Plain X-rays can be used to search for metal fragments, if there is concern about their presence.

6

Electromagnetic radiation – potential bioeffects

During MRI the patient is exposed to three different types of electromagnetic radiation which are potentially hazardous to human tissue:

- the static magnetic field,

- the gradient magnetic fields used for image localisation,

- the RF electromagnetic fields used to generate images and to manipulate the proton nuclei in different imaging sequences.

If applied at sufficiently high levels these may cause heating, vertigo, involuntary muscle contraction and even ventricular fibrillation. Exposure limits are set by the National Radiological Protection Board (NRPB). Field strength for clinical use has an upper limit of 2.0 T, gradient varying magnetic fields must be kept at less than 3 T/s and RF must be limited to 2 W/kg over 1 g of tissue and 0.4 W/kg averaged over the whole body. In current practice these are not exceeded.

Monitoring patients in a MRI system

The changing gradient magnetic fields used for image localisation, and the RF currents used to excite the proton nuclei can induce currents and heating in monitoring leads. Induced currents cause interference with monitoring devices, and have resulted in serious burns to the patient. Precautions must be taken to minimise the risks to patients these include:

- Only *MR compatible equipment* in intact condition should be used ('MR compatible' – the device does not harm the patient and has been demonstrated to neither significantly affect the quality of the diagnostic information nor have its operation affected by the MR device).

- All probes and leads not in use should be removed from the patient.

- Cables and sensors should be placed away from the examination area.

- Cables should not form loops within the magnet bore and should be separated from the patient's skin.

- ECG leads should be braided together to minimise loop formation.

Monitoring equipment can also generate RF; for example, liquid crystal display screens may appear to have a continuous display but may actually be turning on and off at high frequency. The generated RF can be conducted through the patient interface connections (e.g. ECG leads) into the imaging environment and can cause distortion of the MR image. If monitoring equipment is positioned outside of the RF screening around the magnet (now usually in the walls of the magnet room), the monitoring leads can act as aerials picking up RF currents in the general environment and conducting them into the imaging area. Monitoring leads entering the magnet room from outside should pass through low pass filters to exclude signal in the range which interferes with the operating frequency of the MR system. MR 'compatible' commercially available monitoring equipment is contained in a RF screened enclosure. Sensors in this type of equipment may also be shielded, for example, to prevent the LED cycling in the pulse oximeter probe from causing further interference.

Main power supplies can carry interference through the RF screen, and monitoring equipment should use an adequately filtered and isolated power source or be run by batteries. Batteries are strongly ferromagnetic, and battery powered monitoring equipment must be very firmly secured within the magnetic field.

Anaesthesia for MRI

Piped medical gases are essential and the installation of an isolated filtered AC power circuit and RF filters will minimise interference from monitoring equipment. Purchase of an MRI-compatible anaesthetic machine and ventilator, and fibre-optic monitoring systems will reduce potential problems. MRI-compatible anaesthetic machines with MRI-compatible ventilators are now made by most of the major manufacturers, these can be sited adjacent to the magnet bore minimising the length of breathing systems. Space for resuscitation, induction and recovery from anaesthesia will enhance patient safety and increase patient throughput.

In my opinion (C.J. Peden) patients are best anaesthetised outside the magnet room and then transferred into the magnet suite once they are stable and their airway has been secured. The airway of a patient whose head goes first into the magnet is completely inaccessible; in addition, a 'receiver coil' is placed around the area being examined which in the case of a head scan reduces space for tubes and connections. All connections must be plastic. The laryngeal mask is widely used for MRI, and a mask with no ferromagnetic components is specifically made for MRI.

Anaesthetists who have not worked in the MRI environment will be surprised by the level of noise generated during an examination. The gradient magnetic fields produce a loud thumping or tapping which can be very disconcerting for the awake patient, and may necessitate deeper levels of sedation or anaesthesia than might otherwise be required.

Anaesthesia can be maintained with a volatile agent or intravenously. The motor of infusion pumps may start to malfunction at field strengths of 30–50 G, and extended infusion lines are required.

Intensive care patients

MRI shows much greater detail of the central nervous system than CT. Therefore, imaging requests for adult and neonatal intensive care patients with neurological problems are increasing. It is possible to examine these patients with MRI but it needs planning and plenty of time. The main problems are caused by the number of lines and infusion pumps attached to the patient. These should be disconnected unless absolutely essential. Those infusions that must be continued need extensions of adequate length to keep the pumps outside the 30-G line.

Another potential problem with sick infants is maintenance of body temperature as the MR environment is cold and air conditioned to ensure optimal system function. Infants should be returned immediately, at the end of the examination, to a transport incubator.

Micro-shock

There is a theoretical risk of micro-shock being induced by the passage of conducting fluid such as 0.9% saline, through central venous or pulmonary artery catheters in contact with heart muscle in critically ill patients, or by the induction of current in intravascular pacing wires. This possibility has been investigated in an animal model and there appears to be little risk to patients with a central venous catheter. Epicardial pacing wires are potentially unsafe and should be removed if MRI is essential. There has been a report of a pulmonary artery catheter with a thermistor wire that melted during MRI! All patients referred for MRI procedures with cardiovascular catheters and accessories that have internally or externally positioned conductive wires or similar components should not undergo MRI, unless the catheter is removed, due mainly to the risk of excessive heating in the wires.

Conclusion

Anaesthesia and monitoring in the MRI suite needs to be maintained to the same standards as expected in the operating theatre. Extra challenges are produced by the environment of the radiology department and additionally by the unique nature of the MRI suite.

Patient and staff may be endangered by the missile effect of ferromagnetic attraction on every-day objects as well as equipment and surgical implants. Implanted electronic devices may malfunction at very low magnetic field strength, serious burns may result from currents induced in monitoring leads and micro-shock may be induced in intravascular or epicardial devices.

The magnetic, RF and gradient fields may cause artefact and interference with monitoring devices, especially ECG and pulse oximetry.

These challenges are overcome by meticulous attention to detail, the design of RF screened MRI suites and the use of commercial monitoring systems developed specifically for the MRI environment which are both safe for patients and do not distort or degrade the images produced.

References

1. Recommendations for Standards of Monitoring during Anaesthesia and Recovery. Association of Anaesthetists of Great Britain and Ireland, 2000.
2. Sedation and Anaesthesia in Radiology. Report of Joint Working Party of the Royal College of Anaesthetists and the Royal College of Radiologists, 1992.
3. Implementing and Ensuring Safe Sedation Practice for Healthcare Procedures in Adults. Academy of Medical Royal Colleges, 2001.
4. Intensive Care Society Guidelines for the Transport of the Critically Ill Adult, 2002.
5. C.J. Peden. Monitoring patients during anaesthesia for radiological procedures. Current Opinions in Anaesthesiology 1999; 12: 405–410.
6. Association of Anaesthetists. Guidelines for the Provision of Anaesthetic Services in Magnetic Resonance Units, 2002.

MRI: case illustrations

Question 1

55-year-old female.

Long history of unilateral tinitus, deafness, and now ataxia.

Below is a T1-weighted coronal image of the head before and following IV gadolinium (Figs 6.2 and 6.3).

■ From where is this lesion arising?

■ What is the diagnosis?

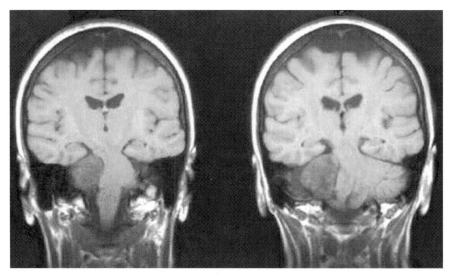

Fig. 6.2 Quiz case.

6

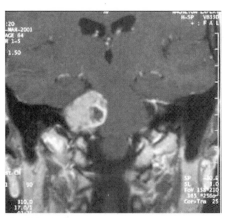
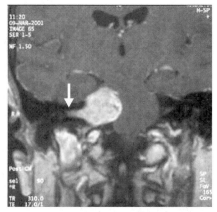

Fig. 6.3 Quiz case.

Answer

Acoustic neuroma

This lesion appears to arise within the right internal auditory canal (arrow) and bulges into the cerebellopontine angle. There is compression of the cerebellum and midline shift to the left. The lesion is very well circumscribed, and enhances intensely following IV gadolinium. The appearances are characteristic of an acoustic neuroma, of which this is a very large example.

Comment

Acoustic neuromas typically have this 'ice cream cone' appearance as they emerge from the internal auditory canal seen well on the axial images (Figs 6.4 and 6.5), and this appearance helps to differentiate them from

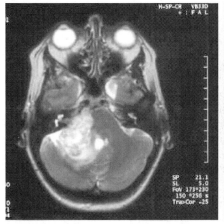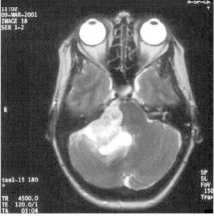

Fig. 6.4 Acoustic neuroma axial T2-weighted image. The tumour is of high signal. Note, the high signal from the CSF identifying it as a T2-weighted image.

6

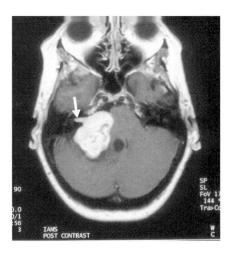

Fig. 6.5 Acoustic neuroma axial post-gadolinium. Note, how the tumour grows along the internal auditary meatus – one of the characteristic signs of acoustic neuroma.

271

meningiomas of the cerebellopontine angle. Acoustic neuromas (85%) arise from the vestibular portion of the eigth cranial nerve and 15% from the cochlear division. They may be sporadic, typically occurring in middle age, or associated with type 2 neurofibromatosis. They are slow growing but may eventually cause facial sensory loss, weakness, ataxia, long tract signs and hydrocephalus due to compression of the fourth ventricle.

Question 2

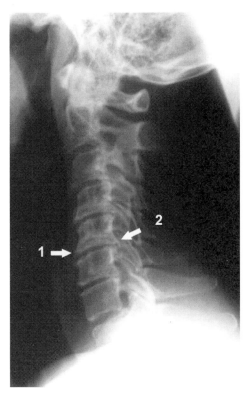

68-year-old female.
During assessment for a general anaesthetic she reports a painful, stiff neck.
On examination, neck movement is severely restricted and precipitates pain and paraesthesia in the right arm.
A lateral cervical spine X-ray and MRI scan of the neck were performed.

■ What are the plain film (Fig. 6.6) findings?

■ What additional information does the MR image (Fig. 6.7) provide?

Fig. 6.6 Quiz case.

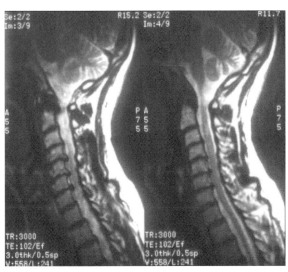

Fig. 6.7 Quiz case.

273

Answer

Degenerative cervical spondylosis with spinal stenosis

The plain film shows reduced intervertebral disc heights from C4 to C7, there are small anterior osteophytes of the C3 to C7 vertebral bodies (Fig. 6.6) [arrow 1]. There are large posterior osteophytes at the C5/C6 level [arrow 2].

The sagittal T2-weighted image (Fig. 6.7) shows narrow dehydrated discs at multiple levels. There are low signal (black) disc protrusions posteriorly most marked at the C5/C6 level. These represent bulging degenerate discs, together with osteophytes from the margins of adjacent vertebral bodies.

There is narrowing of the spinal canal at the C5/C6 level, with obliteration of the subarachnoid space (containing high signal cerebrospinal fluid) and impingement upon the spinal cord. This should also be confirmed with axial images.

Comment

Degenerative disease of the cervical spine can cause stenosis of the nerve root foramina and, less commonly, the spinal canal (particularly in those people with a congenitally narrow canal) due to a combination of several factors (see below). Degenerative disease of the cervical spine or osteoarthritic changes are referred to as cervical spondylosis. Changes include:

- bulging intervertebral discs,

- vertebral end-plate osteophytes,

- ligamentum flavum 'hypertrophy' (the ligament buckles due to osteoarthritis of the underlying facet joints).

Spinal canal and nerve root foraminal stenosis is well shown on MRI, abnormal high signal may be seen within the spinal cord on T2-weighted images, if there is actual cord compression. Classically, nerve root compression causes pain, paraesthesiae and lower motor neurone signs in the upper limbs. Spinal cord compression causes a myelopathy with additional upper motor neurone signs below the level of impingement, and sometimes urinary symptoms.

6

Question 3

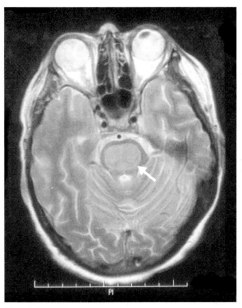

50-year-old male.
7-day history of gastroenteritis. He was severely dehydrated and confused.
Plasma sodium = 120 mmol/L. Hypertonic saline was given to correct it; 24 hours later, he developed flaccid weakness in all four limbs, and difficulty in swallowing.
Below is a T2-weighted axial image of the brain (Fig. 6.8).

■ What is the abnormality?

■ What conditions are associated with this diagnosis?

■ What is the prognosis?

Fig. 6.8 Quiz case.

Answer

Central pontine myelinolysis
There is a large oval-shaped area of high signal within the pons (arrow). This represents demyelination. This is central pontine myelinolysis. This is a rare condition in which there is massive demyelination involving the pons and sometimes the basal ganglia, thalami and internal capsule.
Signs include cranial nerve palsies (particularly the fourth, fifth and sixth), pyramidal signs in the limbs, bulbar signs and coma.

Associated conditions
■ Hyponatraemia, which is rapidly corrected.

■ Chronic alcoholism.

■ Chronic liver disease.

The prognosis is poor – the 6-month survival rate is approximately 10% and residual neurological deficits are common. In this case, CPM may have been avoided by giving 0.9% saline as the initial resuscitation fluid, with frequent electrolyte analysis, aiming to correct the hyponatraemia by no more than 10–12 mmol/L in 24 hours.

Question 4

28-year-old pregnant female with hyperemesis gravidarum.
Persistent vomiting and dehydration over the past 36 hours.
Severe headache and now some left-sided weakness.
Shown below are a proton-density weighted axial image of the brain
(Fig. 6.9), and a sagittal MRV image (Fig. 6.10).

■ What is the diagnosis?

■ Name some predisposing factors.

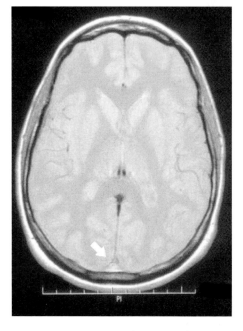

Fig. 6.9 Quiz case.

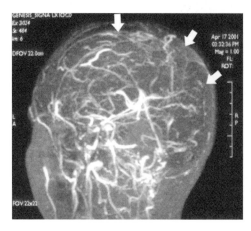

6

Fig. 6.10 Quiz case (arrows).

Answer

Superior sagittal sinus thrombosis

The axial image shows high signal thrombus within the superior sagittal sinus posteriorly (arrow) (Fig. 6.9), where flowing blood would normally produce a 'flow-void' as in the normal T2-weighted image (Fig. 6.11). The MRV image shows a lack of signal in the expected position of the superior sagittal sinus (arrows) (Fig. 6.10). A further case of sinus thrombosis on MRV (transverse sinus thrombosis) is demonstrated in Fig. 6.12.

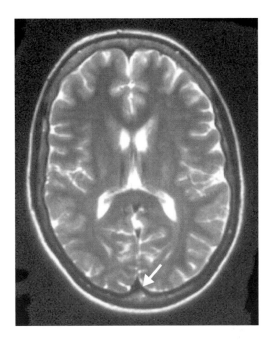

Fig. 6.11 Normal – flow-void coming from the sagittal sinus (arrow).

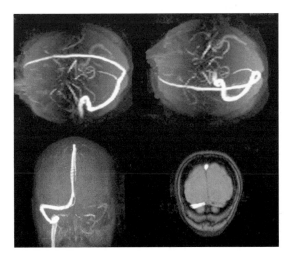

Fig. 6.12 Transverse sinus thrombosis MRV.

Predisposing factors

- Pregnancy.

- Oral contraceptive.

- Thrombophilia.

- Dehydration.

- Systemic malignancy, e.g. childhood leukaemia.

- Sinusitis and other local sepsis.

- Intracranial tumours, e.g. meningioma.

Comment

Intracranial sinus thrombosis may also be diagnosed with contrast enhanced CT, however, MRI is the investigation of choice when the diagnosis is suspected. It is sensitive, and non-invasive – in contrast to conventional cerebral angiography.

Presenting symptoms include headache, seizures, focal neurological deficits and coma. Sinus thrombosis may lead to venous infarction, haemorrage and cerebral oedema.

Question 5

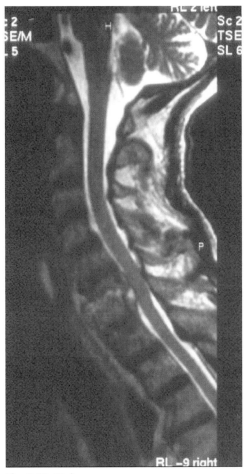

36-year-old intravenous drug user.
Long history of neck pain, malaise and low grade fever. Below is a T2-weighted sagittal image of the cervical spine (Fig. 6.13).

- What is the cause for this patient's symptoms?

- What other groups are at risk of this condition?

Fig. 6.13 Quiz case.

Answer

Discitis with epidural abscess
An area of high signal (white) is seen within the C6/C7 disc space, representing fluid and inflammatory change. There is destruction of the end plates of the C6 and C7 vertebral bodies, which are reduced in height. Some high signal is seen bulging posteriorly (arrow) into the anterior epidural space – this is an epidural abscess.

Groups at risk of spinal infection
Children – haematogenous spread of infection to a vertebral body or a vascularised intervertebral disc; usually in the lumbar spine.

Adults

- Intravenous drug users.
- Diabetic.
- Immunosupression, e.g. steroids.
- Alcoholics.
- Genito-urinary infections and instrumentation.
- Post-spinal surgery.

Infection starts as a vertebral osteomyelitis which then 'ruptures' into the disc space. May occur at any level, but most commonly lumbar spine.

Comment

Epidural abscess usually occurs as a complication of vertebral osteomyelitis or discitis, as in this case, and may cause nerve root or spinal cord compression. Prior to the era of MRI, diagnosis was by the invasive technique of myelography. Spinal infection may also spread anteriorly, leading to a retropharyngeal abscess in the cervical region, or psoas abscess in the lumbar spine (see Fig. 6.14). The condition is a neurosurgical emergency frequently requiring surgical drainage, decompression and stabilisation to prevent spinal cord infarction.

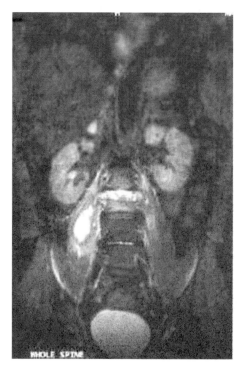

Fig. 6.14 Lumbar discitis and psoas abscess. Coronal STIR image sequence, this is a fat suppression sequence in which pathology usually appears high signal. In this example, the lumbar intervertebral disc and both adjacent vertebral bodies are of high signal. There is an abscess extending into the right psoas muscle.

Question 6

40-year-old male.
Progressive left-sided weakness, visual loss and generalised seizures.
Below are T2-weighted images of the brain (Figs 6.15 and 6.16).

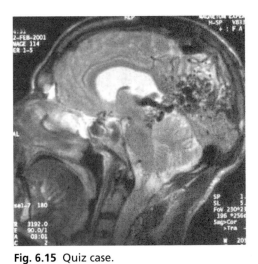

- What is the nature of the this lesion?
- What is the diagnosis?

Fig. 6.15 Quiz case.

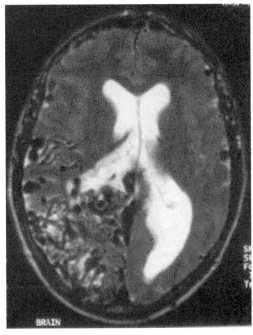

Fig. 6.16 Quiz case.

Answer

Arteriovenous malformation

There are multiple areas of serpiginous 'flow-voids', predominantly in the right parieto-occipital region. These are extremely extensive and represent dilated vessels. There is some associated cerebral atrophy with compensatory mild dilation of the cerebral ventricles.

Comment

Arteriovenous malformations (AVMs) are congenital lesions, which may be multiple and can progressively increase in size. Patients may present with symptoms of a space-occupying lesion such as headache, focal neurological deficits and epilepsy. AVMs are also a cause of subarachnoid and intracranial haemorrage. Conventional angiography may still be indicated in cases where surgery or percutaneous embolisation is being considered, in order to more clearly define the feeding arteries and draining veins.

Interventional procedures: case illustrations

Anaesthetic support is occasionally required for patients undergoing interventional procedures in the radiology department; anaesthetic input is likely to increase as the procedures grow ever complex. The number and diversity of radiological procedures are increasing with improved imaging technology and better interventional techniques and devices. There are vast number of conditions and pathologies which now require interventional radiology input at either the stage of diagnosis or treatment.

Most intervention is performed using fluoroscopy, CT or ultrasound image guidance (ultrasound dealt with in Chapter 7 – Ultrasound and intensive care). MRI intervention is performed in some centres, but it accounts for only a small proportion of cases performed. It requires a specialised open MRI scanner and non-feromagnetic equipment, the high demand on MRI scanners also limits its use. Anaesthetists require a working knowledge of common interventional procedures, the common complications and a working knowledge regarding radiation protection as both CT and fluoroscopy use ionising radiation.

The following cases serve to illustrate some of the more common interventional procedures and their potential complications.

Question 7

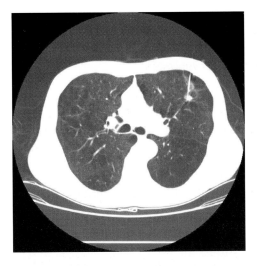

Fig. 6.17 Quiz case.

- What is this procedure (Figs 6.17 and 6.18)?

- What complication has occurred?

- What are the contraindications?

- What are the potential complications?

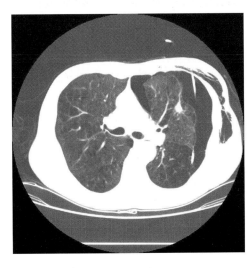

Fig. 6.18 Quiz case.

Answer

CT-guided lung biopsy complicated by pneumothorax (Table 6.1)

Prior to lung biopsy, patients should have a platelet count (above 50,000) and prothrombin time (INR less than 1.3) performed. Antiplatelet drugs should be discontinued for 7 days prior to the procedure. Resuscitation equipment should be readily available including chest drain or a pleur-evac device. Patients should have a venous line in place and are monitored with an oxygen saturation monitor. Oxygen may be administered during the procedure – if a pneumothorax develops, oxygen is more rapidly absorbed than air.

Table 6.1 Contraindications to lung biopsy

---

1. Patient with single lung (unable to tolerate small pneumothorax).

2. Severe COPD.

3. Mechanical ventilation (increased pneumothorax risk).

4. Bullae in vicinity of lesion to be biopsied.

5. Vascular lesion – AVM.

6. Pulmonary artery hypertension.

7. Bleeding disorder.

Patients are positioned supine or prone prior to localising the lesion for biopsy with CT. Subcutaneous structures are infiltrated with local anaesthetic (being careful not to transgress the pleura with the local anaesthetic needle). A fine needle aspiration biopsy (20 or 22 gauge) or core biopsy can be performed. The needle is advanced to the edge of the lesion. This may be introduced alone or as part of a coaxial system. Samples should be performed in arrested respiration. Cytopathology support during the procedure is preferable. In addition to aspiration samples, some centres perform core biopsy. The biopsy site should be placed in a dependent position following the procedure as this promotes atelectasis and reduces alveolar size – it may help prevent pneumothorax by tamponading the puncture site.

Using a 20- or 22-gauge needle, sensitivities of up to 90% can be achieved for thoracic malignancy.

Complications

1. *Pneumothorax* (see Fig. 6.18): For FNAB, the risk is approximately 5–15%. Emphysematous changes, multiple pleural punctures, core biopsies and positive pressure ventilation all increase the risk of pneumothorax.

2. *Haemorrhage*: Haemoptysis may occur, this is usually self-limiting.

3. Air embolus has been described.

Patients should be monitored (pulse, blood pressure, oxygen saturations for 4 hours) prior to discharge. Many centres perform a chest X-ray to exclude pneumothorax prior to discharge.

Question 8

58-year-old patient with a 3-week history of back pain and jaundice. ERCP was attempted but it was not possible to access the common bile duct.

▪ What procedure has been performed (Figs 6.19 and 6.20)?

▪ How is this device deployed?

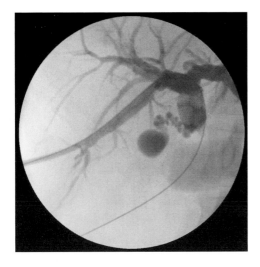

Fig. 6.19 Quiz case.

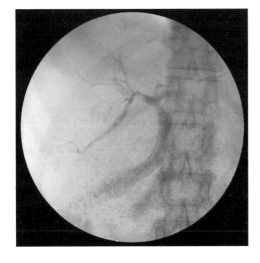

Fig. 6.20 Quiz case.

Answer

Percutaneous transhepatic cholangiogram and biliary stent

A percutaneous transhepatic cholangiogram (PTC) is performed in cases of biliary obstruction when ERCP is not possible (previous Bilroth II gastrectomy, choledochojejunostomy) or if ERCP has failed. A fine needle (22 guage) is used to puncture the biliary tree and inject radiographic contrast in order to demonstrate the anatomy of the dilated bile ducts. This initial puncture can be performed under fluoroscopy or using ultrasound guidance (when a specific duct is targeted). From the cholangiogram, it is usually possible to confirm the cause of bile duct obstruction. Common causes included gallstones, cholangio carcinoma, pancreatic carcinoma, extrinsic compression from liver metastases or benign strictures, e.g. after bile duct surgery. Metallic stents are inserted only for malignant bile duct strictures/obstruction.

In order to deploy a metal stent, it is necessary to position a guide wire across the bile duct stricture and into the duodenum. This is sometimes done using the initial access for the PTC or it may be performed by repuncturing the biliary tree at a more suitable site. Once a guide wire is in the duodenum, the stricture can be dilated with a balloon catheter (especially if very tight), prior to deploying the stent. The stent delivery system is passed over the previously sited guide wire and deployed with its tip just into the duodenum. If a catheter is inserted along the guide wire, a check cholangiogram can be performed to confirm patency and position (see Fig. 6.20). The advantage of internal biliary drainage is that it avoids the electrolyte and fluid losses, and risk of sepsis associated with external drainage.

6

Question 9

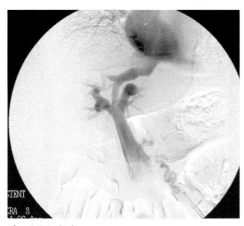

Fig. 6.21 Quiz case.

53-year-old man.
Hepatitis C positive for 16 years following a blood transfusion.
Bleeding oesophageal varices.

- What is the therapeutic intervention that has been performed (Figs 6.21–6.23)?
- What are the indications for this procedure?
- What are the complications?

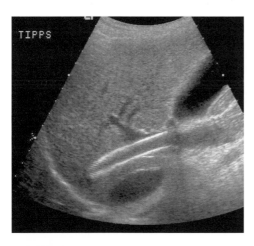

Fig. 6.22 Quiz case.

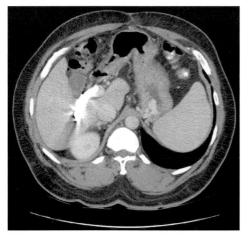

Fig. 6.23 Quiz case.

Answer

Transjugular intra-hepatic porto-systemic shunt

Surgical porto-systemic shunts have been created in the past to treat portal hypertension, e.g. portocaval or splenorenal shunts. A similar result can now be achieved less invasively using transjugular intra-hepatic porto-systemic shunt (TIPS). This involves forming an artificial channel between a hepatic vein and an intrahepatic branch of the portal vein (Table 6.2).

Procedure

Using a cutaneous approach, a communication tract is created between a hepatic vein and the portal vein to decompress portal hypertension.

The hepatic veins are catheterised using the right internal jugular vein for access (via the SVC and right atrium). A passage is created from the hepatic vein into the portal vein through liver parenchyma. Direct measurement of the systemic and the portal pressures is then made. The tract is then dilated with a balloon. A metallic stent is deployed in order to try and maintain the tract against the recoil of the surrounding liver parenchyma. The resultant reduction in portal venous pressure can then be measured. In general, a gradient of less than 12 mmHg is the target. Serial dilations of the stent can be performed until satisfactory pressure levels have been reached. Varices can be embolised at this stage (if required) using a catheter passing through the stent into the portal veins for access. In patients who may go on to liver transplantation, the stent should occupy less than half of the extrahepatic portal vein.

Complications of TIPS

- Technical failure or incorrect positioning.

- Shunt failure/obstruction (resulting in rebleeding from varices).

- Encephalopathy.

- Hepatic injury.

Table 6.2 Indications for TIPS

- Acute variceal haemorrhage

- Recurrent variceal haemorrhage

- Portal hypertensive gastropathy

- Intractable ascites

- Hepatic chylothorax

- Budd–Chiari syndrome

Cirrhosis and portal hypertension

The commonest cause of portal hypertension is cirrhosis secondary to alcoholic liver disease or chronic hepatitis B or C (see Fig. 6.24), further causes are listed in Table 6.3. Imaging features of cirrhosis and portal hypertension include liver nodularity, reversal of portal blood flow (demonstrated on ultrasound), porto-systemic colateral vessels, splenomegaly, ascites and complications such as hepatoma. Porto-systemic colateral vessels occur at many sites (see Table 6.4) as a consequence of portal hypertension (see Fig. 6.25).

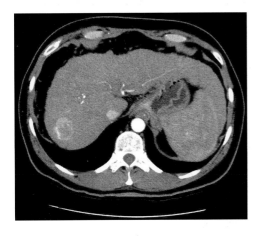

Fig. 6.24 Liver cirrhosis complicated by hepatoma. The liver has an irregular, nodular outline which is typical of cirrhosis. Hepatomas, such as this example, have avid arterial enhancement.

Table 6.3 Causes of Portal Hypertension

- Prehepatic
  - Portal vein compression/thrombosis

- Hepatic
  - Cirrhosis (Fig. 6.24)
  - Hepatic fibrosis congenital/acquired
  - Cystic fibrosis
  - Chronic malaria
  - Schistosomiasis

- Post-hepatic
  - Budd–Chiari syndrome
  - Constrictive pericarditis

Table 6.4 **Sites of porto-systemic collaterals**

- Oesophageal

- Coronary vein

- Para-umbilical

- Abdominal wall

- Perisplenic (Fig. 6.25)

- Splenorenal

- Gastric

- Mesenteric

- Haemorrhoidal

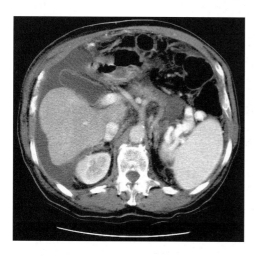

Fig. 6.25 Hepatitis C cirrhosis complicated by portal hypertension. There is a moderate volume of ascites and dramatic varices at the splenic hilum.

Question 10

■ What procedure has been carried out?

■ What are the indications and what are the common complications (Fig. 6.26)?

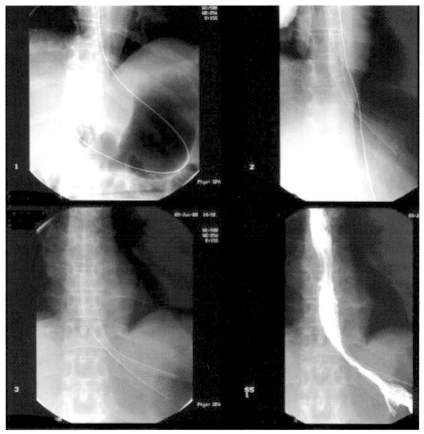

Fig. 6.26 Quiz case.

Answer

Oesophageal stent

There is a metallic oesophageal stent which has been inserted in the lower oesophagus. Malignant oesophageal strictures (whether due to intrinsic or extrinsic compression) are the main indication (stents are not indicated for benign disease). Stents are either uncovered, i.e. metal mesh only, or covered with a plastic membrane over the mesh – covered stents. Covered stents can be used to treat malignant oesophageal fistulae. Retrosternal pain can be quite troublesome for few days after stent placement and

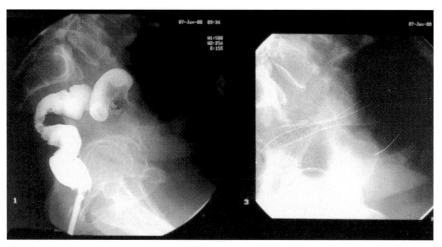

Fig. 6.27 Colo-rectal stent. The initial image shows a narrow irregular stricture at the junction of the recto-sigmoid colon. The second image is of the metallic stent once in position.

powerful analgesia is often required. Profound gastro-oesophageal reflux usually occurs and anti-reflux medication or acid suppression therapy (proton pump inhibitors, etc.) needs to be prescribed. It is often helpful to elevate the head of the bed. Bolus obstruction can occur and fizzy drinks should be taken following meals to help clear any food debris from around the stent. Tumour ingrowth (particularly with uncovered stents) can be a problem leading to restenosis or occlusion. Covered stents have a membrane over the meshwork to help prevent this happening, although they are more prone to migration. Other complications include oesophageal perforation and stent migration.

Colo-rectal stenting can also be performed, (see Fig. 6.27). This is useful in cases of large bowel obstruction as a definitive palliative procedure or as a temporising measure prior to colonic surgery. The stent decompresses the large bowel obstruction so that elective surgery is possible after formal bowel preparation and work-up. The stent is then removed at surgery with the diseased bowel.

6

Question 11

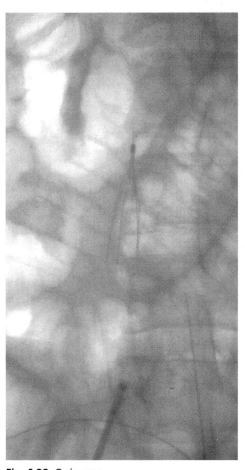

■ What is this device (Fig. 6.28)?

Fig. 6.28 Quiz case.

6

Answer

IVC filter

Pulmonary embolism is a significant cause of morbidity and mortality. Normally patients with DVT or PE are treated with anticoagulation therapy. As many as 20% of patients will have recurrent thrombo embolic events. The purpose of IVC filters is to prevent thrombi generated in the pelvic veins and lower limbs embolising to the right side of the heart and into the pulmonary circulation (Fig. 6.29). Ideally, highly efficient filtration without impedance of blood flow is required (Table 6.5).

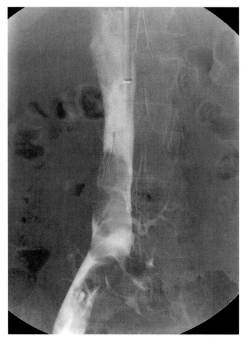

Fig. 6.29 IVC filter note abundant clot proximal to it.

Table 6.5 **Indications for IVC filters**

Accepted indications
1. Contraindication to anticoagulation
2. Complication of anticoagulation
3. Failure of anticoagulation recurrent PE or inability to achieve adequate anticoagulation
4. Massive PE with residual DVT in patient at risk of further PE

Further indications
1. Severe trauma without documented PE or DVT; closed head injury, spinal cord injury, multiple long bone or pelvic fractures
2. High-risk patients, intensive care patients

Placement
Puncture of the right internal jugular vein or common femoral vein is performed to obtain access to the IVC. A catheter is advanced to the proximal IVC and a cavagram is performed (Fig. 6.30) to assess the level of the renal veins, accessory renal veins and possible caval abnormalities. The diameter of the cava is measured as dilation can predispose to caval filter migration. The dilivery system is introduced via a sheath to a level just below the renal veins or accessory renal veins, if present. The filter is

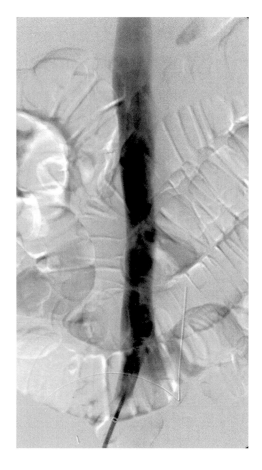

Fig. 6.30 Cavagram.

Table 6.6 **Complications of IVC filters**

- Misplacement of filter
- Migration of filter
- Caval penetration
- Filter embolisation
- Caval occlusion

---

deployed at this level after carefully confirming the position relative to the renal veins. Early morbidity is associated with incorrect positioning, above the renal veins or following migration (Table 6.6). Different types of filter exist such as Bird's Nest filter or Greenfield filters. Some removable filters now exist (Fig. 6.31) but caution needs to be exercised in the young adult or paediatric population.

295

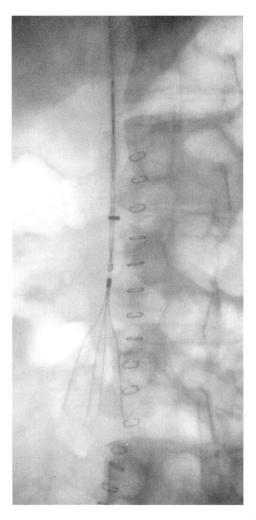

Fig. 6.31 Removable IVC filter.

Question 12

78-year-old man with a 1-day history of altered blood per rectum.
The patient was shocked and hypotensive when admitted.
A CT scan was performed. IV, but *no oral* contrast was given for the scan.

■ What do the CT scans (Figs 6.32–6.35) show?

■ What intervention has been performed?

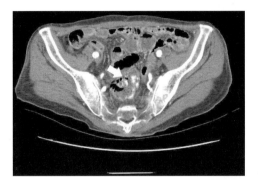

Fig. 6.32 Quiz case.

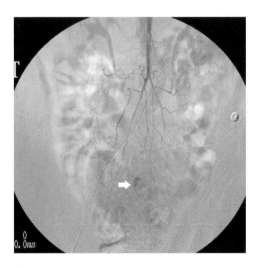

Fig. 6.33 Quiz case.

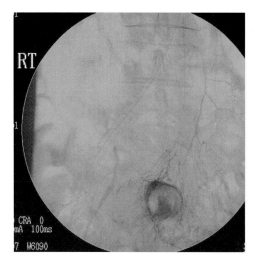

Fig. 6.34 Quiz case.

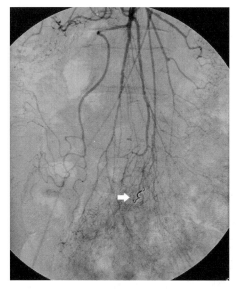

Fig. 6.35 Quiz case.

Answer

Acute gastrointestinal haemorrhage

Melanoma metastasis to small bowel

The CT scan (Fig. 6.32) demonstrates dense contrast in a loop of bowel despite the lack of oral contrast having been given. This is extravasation of IV contrast – active bleeding from a loop of small bowel, there is no mass seen to suggest a tumour and no signs of inflammatory change in the adjacent mesentery.

A superior mesenteric artery arteriogram (Fig. 6.33) was performed and this shows active bleeding from the mid-pelvic region consistent with bleeding coming from the distal jejunum or ileum. A microcatheter was passed further distally (Fig. 6.34) and active bleeding is again seen – contrast passes into the small bowel lumen. The final image of the series (Fig. 6.35) shows embolisation coils, but no evidence of continued active bleeding. The distal position of the coils reduces the chance of small bowel ischaemia. The bleeding lesion was later identified as a melanoma metastasis. Complications from angiography are rare, bleeding from the puncture site is the most common occuring in approximately 3%. (see Table 6.7).

Table 6.7 Complication from angiography

- Systemic
  - Contrast reaction
  - Deterioration in renal function secondary to contrast load

- Puncture site
  - Bleeding
  - Haematoma
  - Pseudoaneurysm formation (Fig. 6.36)
  - Infection

- Vessel
  - Thrombosis/vessel occlusion
  - Embolism of clot or plaque; air embolus
  - Dissection of vessel wall

6

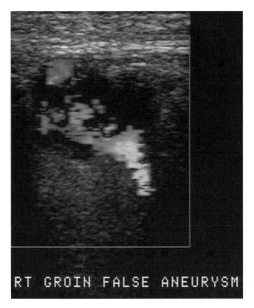

RT GROIN FALSE ANEURYSM

Fig. 6.36 Arterial pseudoaneurysm colour Doppler image. This is a complication of arterial puncture, usually when a large introducer sheath has been used. It is a non-endothelialised space in communication with the artery which contains pulsating arterial blood. Treatment methods include surgery, ultrasound-guided compression which is painful and time consuming or ultrasound-guided thrombin injection.

7

Ultrasound and intensive care

Ultrasound imaging: principles of image formation

Ultrasound is an imaging modality which relies upon the use of sound waves which are transmitted into the body and then reflected back again from the structures being examined. The device which transmits the sound pulses is called a transducer. This contains a piezo-electric crystal which is able to convert electrical signal into sound and then convert the returning sound wave back into electrical signals again. Different reflecting surfaces or interfaces within the body reflect sound to different degrees.

A strong reflector appears as a bright white area (echogenic) on the image, whereas areas from which no echoes have been obtained appear as black (anechoic).

Every ultrasound image is composed of a discrete number of lines of echo data placed side by side to appear continuous. Multiple lines of data are built up as the ultrasound beam sweeps through the field of view. In order to build up each of the single lines of data, the time taken for the returning echo is measured. This allows the depth of the reflecting interface to be determined. Each sweep of the ultrasound beam produces one frame of data (composed of multiple lines). Many complete sweeps are performed every second which produces the frame rate (frames per second). The operation is analogous to the operation of a television camera. At any one moment, the ultrasound beam is scanning along one of the many lines of sight which will ultimately form the image. The image is constantly updated at the prevailing frame rate. This can be frozen and hard copy images produced.

The resolution of the picture produced depends on the wavelength of the sound wave used – this can be varied. There is a trade off between resolution and penetration. Higher frequency transducers allow better resolution, but as the frequency is increased penetration is reduced. As a general rule, the highest frequency transducer should be used to achieve the penetration required.

An ultrasound image is a map of reflectivity of the body part scanned. Organs containing multiple interfaces will produce multiple echoes and this is characteristic of solid organs like liver, spleen and kidneys. Structures containing no interfaces will appear echo-free, such as liquid or urine in the bladder.

Doppler ultrasound

The apparent change in frequency produced by relative movement between a sound emitter and receiver is called the Doppler effect (Christian Doppler 1805–1853). This principle is used in ultrasound systems to provide information about blood flow. This may simply be in the form of audio information, a spectral display or as colour Doppler displays. Two main ways of obtaining Doppler information can be used:

1. Continuous wave ultrasound beam – information presented as either an audio signal and/or a spectral display.

7

2. Pulsed wave ultrasound beams whereby audio, spectral and colour display of data are possible.

Duplex Doppler is a term used to refer to a combination of grey scale and pulsed-Doppler display. This produces a grey scale image with a line of sight along which there is a Doppler acquisition marker/gate. The position and size of the gate can be varied within the ultrasound image, so that it lies within the vessel or area of interest. When the machine is switched into Doppler mode, a real-time Doppler spectral display appears on the monitor. This can be used to assess flow direction, resistance, evidence of spectral broadening and peak velocity.

Colour Doppler and power Doppler

The disadvantage of duplex Doppler is that at any moment in time Doppler information is only being acquired from one single location. Colour Doppler and power Doppler allow detection of flow over a large area of the field of view. Colour Doppler imaging involves assessing a nominated area for evidence of Doppler shifts and then colour coding those regions. It allows assessment to be made of the relative velocity and direction of blood flow. Colour images of moving blood and grey scale images both appear in real time. Power doppler is more sensitive in detecting blood flow but the velocity and direction of flow cannot be assessed.

Clinical applications for the use of Doppler are numerous and include:

- carotid artery assessment (carotid artery stenosis);

- peripheral Doppler venography (deep venous thrombosis);

- assessment of flow in any of the intra-abdominal vessels, e.g.
  - aorta (aneurysm), inferior vena cava (thrombosis),
  - portal veins (direction of flow), hepatic veins (patency), varices,
  - renal arteries (stenosis).

Doppler can be used to assess the vascularity of tissues such as tumours or inflammatory lesions.

7

Applications of ultrasound for patients on intensive care units

Ultrasound imaging has a huge variety of applications for patients on intensive care units. These include both diagnostic and therapeutic applications, some of the more common applications are listed below. Ultrasound is readily portable and can often be performed at short notice. The size of machines, the quality and resolution of images has improved over the last decade. It is a versatile imaging modality with many applications on intensive care units.

Thoracic

Diagnosic applications
- Pleural effusions (see Fig. 7.1).

- Empyema.

- Pleural biopsy.

Therapeutic applications
- Fluid aspiration.

- Chest drain insertion (see Fig. 7.2).

Abdomen

Diagnosic applications
- Biliary disease – gallstones (see Fig. 7.3), bile duct obstruction (see Fig. 7.4), cholecystitis.

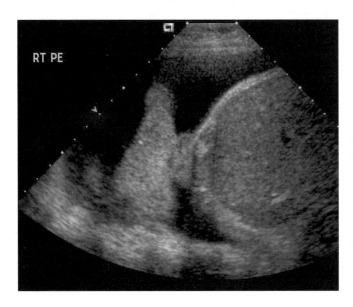

Fig. 7.1 Pleural effusion. The collapsed lung can be seen within the pleural fluid. Fluid is readily identified using ultrasound whether in the pleural space or within the abdomen.

7

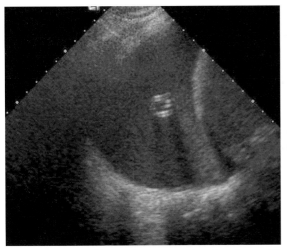

Fig. 7.2 Pleural effusion drainage – pigtail catheter. The insertion of pigtail catheters on intensive care units is performed most safely using ultrasound guidance.

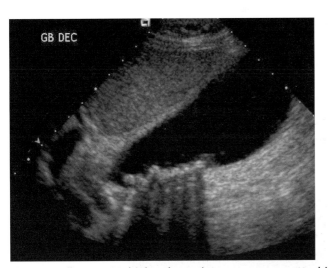

GB DEC

Fig. 7.3 Gallstones. Multiple echogenic stones are present which cast an acoustic shadow posteriorly. The demonstration of gallstones on intensive care units can be important in cases of obstructive jaundice, cholecystitis and pancreatitis.

- Pancreatic disease and its complications, e.g. pancreatitis and pseudocysts (see Fig. 7.5).

- Renal disease – stones, hydronephrosis (see Fig. 7.6), parenchymal thickness, etc.

- Bowel pathology – appendicitis (see Figs 7.7 and 7.8).

- Abdominal trauma – solid organ injury with free fluid (Fig. 7.9), ascites (Fig. 7.10).

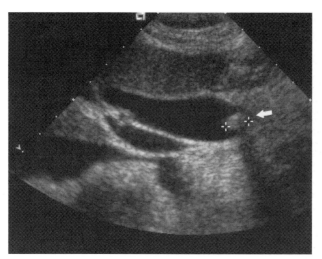

Fig. 7.4 Dilated bile duct. The diameter of the duct can be accurately measured with ultrasound and in cases of obstruction, the cause may be identified such as this gallstone. Duct size increases with age or following cholecystectomy.

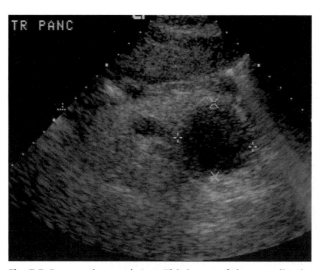

Fig. 7.5 Pancreatic pseudocyst. This is one of the complications of pancreatitis which is readily diagnosed on ultrasound. If the collections become infected, then ultrasound-guided drainage is appropriate. Sterile collections do not usually require drainage.

7

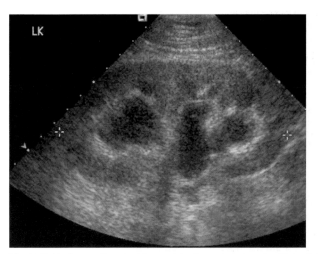

Fig. 7.6 Hydronephrosis. The pelvicalyceal system is dilated. Proximal causes of obstruction such as proximal calculi can be diagnosed on ultrasound; the ureters are, however, poorly seen except the distal few centimetres at the vesicoureteric junction.

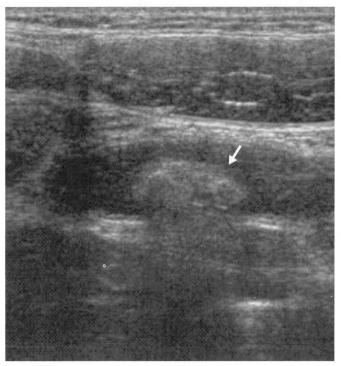

Fig. 7.7 Appendicitis. Ultrasound has poor sensitivity but high specificity in the diagnosis of appendicitis. Features include a 'lith', (arrow) a blind ending, non-compressible loop of bowel 6 mm or greater in diameter and surrounding fluid.

7

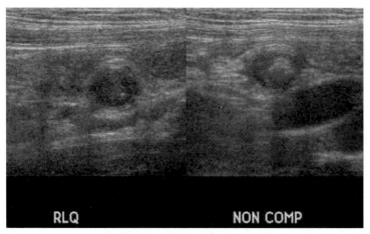

Fig. 7.8 Appendicitis. Images in transverse section demonstrating failure of compression of the appendix.

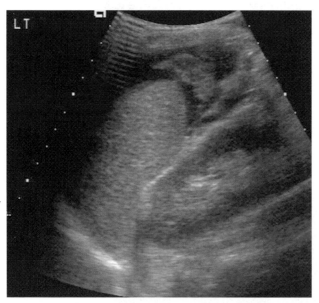

Fig. 7.9 Free fluid from splenic trauma. Ultrasound is extremely sensitive in the identification of free fluid. In the setting of trauma, the *absence* of free fluid is very useful in excluding intra-peritoneal haemorrhage. It has largely replaced diagnostic peritoneal lavage (DPL).

Therapeutic applications

- Gall bladder drainage.

- Pseudocyst/ascitic drainage.

- Abscess drainage (see Figs 7.11 and 7.12).

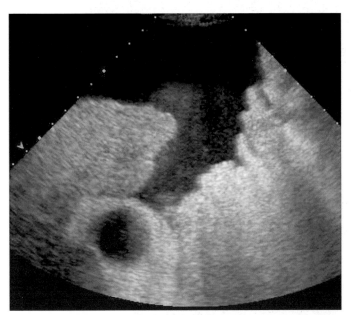

Fig. 7.10 Abdominal ascites. The anechoic fluid is readily visualised in this patient with chronic liver disease.

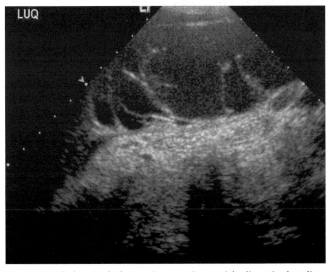

Fig. 7.11 Abdominal abscess in a patient with diverticular disease.

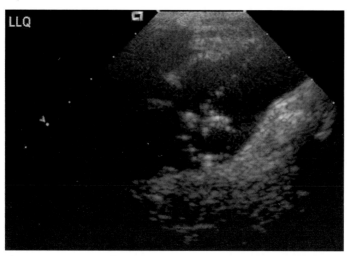

Fig. 7.12 Drainage of abdominal abscess. Ultrasound is the imaging modality of choice for the drainage of suitable abdominal abscesses. Real-time visualisation is possible for the insertion of pigtail drains – which are well seen on ultrasound. This is a portable technique which can be used on intensive care units.

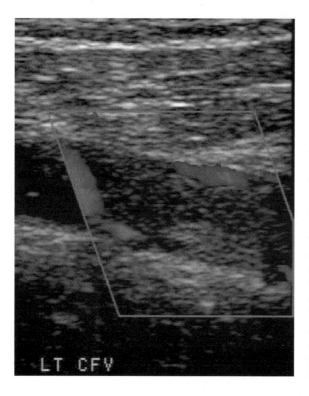

Fig. 7.13 DVT.
A combination of grey scale ultrasound and Doppler ultrasound is used in the diagnosis of deep vein thrombosis. A normal vein can be compressed, it demonstrates phasic flow in time with respiration and squeezing on the limb augments blood flow. Deep vein thrombosis interrupts flow and prevents complete compression of the vein. The clot is frequently directly visualised. The technique is eminently suitable for patients on intensive care units, many of whom are at high risk of DVT.

7

Vascular: arterial and venous

Diagnosic applications
- Ischaemic limbs.

- Deep vein thrombosis (upper and lower limbs) (see Fig. 7.13).

Therapeutic applications
- Guided insertion of internal jugular lines.

Musculoskeletal

Diagnosic applications
- Septic arthropathy.

Therapeutic applications
- Joint aspiration.

Ultrasound can be used to guide an extremely wide range of procedures including guided central line insertion, pleural aspiration, marking sites for safe insertion of chest drains, solid organ or tumour biopsy and various abdominal work. There are several advantages of ultrasound over other forms of imaging, which make it extremely useful for sick or ventilated patients and especially those with numerous support tubes and patients on intensive care units who cannot be moved (Table 7.1).

Table 7.1 **Advantages and disadvantages of ultrasound**

Advantages
1. Portable – patients need not be moved
2. No ionising radiation
3. Imaging is in real time so allowance can be made for patient movement or breathing during interventional procedures
4. Imaging is not restricted to fixed planes, e.g. sagital, coronal

Disadvantages
1. Small field of view
2. Image quality is restricted in large obese patients
3. Bowel gas impairs image quality
4. Ultrasound is operator dependent and requires specialist training

---

7

Ultrasound imaging: case illustrations

Question 1

47-year-old Female.
Requires central line insertion. Neck ultrasound. Transverse plane.

■ Name the structures in the image (Figs 7.14 and 7.15).

■ Briefly outline how ultrasound can be used to guide central line insertion.

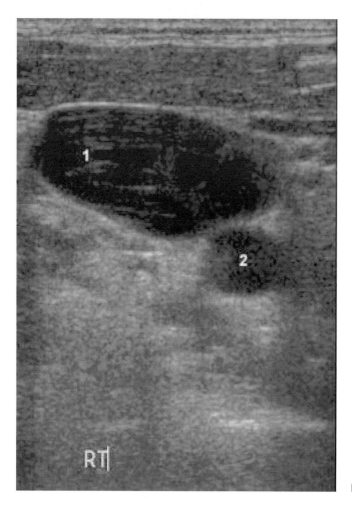

Fig. 7.14 Quiz case.

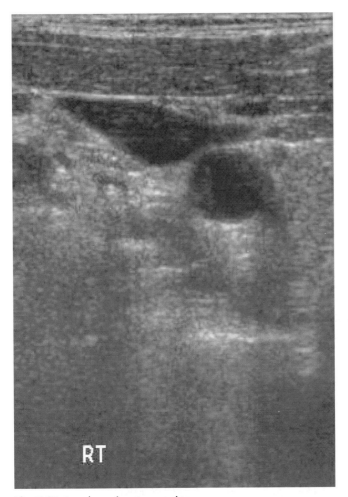

Fig. 7.15 Jugular vein compression.

Answer

Ultrasound guidance central line insertion

The internal jugular vein (No. 1) and the common carotid artery (No. 2) are adjacent structures in the neck. US image guidance is invaluable when inserting jugular venous central lines.

A high frequency linear or curvilinear probe should be selected. If no previous lines have been inserted, the right side is generally chosen as this is the larger vein with a more direct course to the SVC. Scanning the neck will identify the course of the jugular, confirm patency, the relationship to the carotid and assess whether there are any intervening structures such as lymph nodes. The jugular is thin walled, its calibre varies with respiration and it can be occluded with mild compression. The carotid is smaller, thick walled, and can be seen pulsating. The carotid cannot be occluded with mild pressure. Once the internal jugular is identified using these criteria, then a puncture site can be chosen and a mark made on the skin superficial to this.

The skin is then cleansed with antiseptic solution and local anaesthetic infiltrated. The jugular is then punctured using a introducer needle (18 gauge) and blood is aspirated into a connected syringe to confirm a venous puncture. The puncture is performed under direct US visualisation. It should be possible to follow the needle tip from the subcutaneous layers into the vein. Introducer kits vary but most comprise a guide wire which is inserted via the initial needle. The introducer needle is then withdrawn leaving the guide wire. The central line is then inserted over the guide wire. Air embolus is a theoretical complication when the system is open to the atmosphere, e.g. withdrawing the wire. This should be done in arrested respiration where possible.

Complications of line insertion include carotid puncture and haematoma formation in the soft tissues of the neck (see Fig. 7.16). Ultrasound should reduce the incidence of these complications.

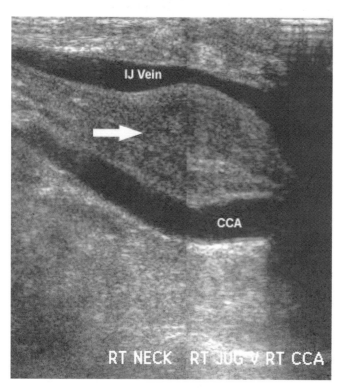

Fig. 7.16 Failed jugular line insertion. There is a large haematoma (arrow) compressing the internal jugular vein.

Question 2

32-year-old male. Multiple lymph nodes in neck.

▪ What is this procedure (Fig. 7.17)?

▪ What are the main complications?

▪ What are the contraindications?

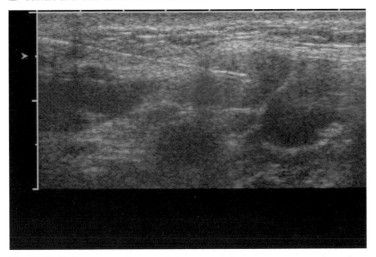

Fig. 7.17 Quiz case.

Answer

Ultrasound-guided biopsy

Needle biopsies can be divided into two basis types – fine needle aspiration biopsy (FNAB) and core biopsy. FNAB uses a small gauge needle, usually 22 gauge, which is inserted into the lesion requiring biopsy under ultrasound visualisation. A syringe is connected to the needle and suction (10 ml) is applied whilst the needle tip is repeatedly inserted and withdrawn through (the edge of) the lesion. If a large tumour is being sampled, then the edge of the lesion is often most likely to yield diagnostic material as the lesion centre may be necrotic. The sample is then spread on slides prior to cytological examination. FNAB can generally only be used for cytology and not histology. FNAB is often used for targeted biopsy of head and neck masses, focal liver masses or where neoplasia is suspected. The small calibre of the needle means that bleeding complications are rare.

Core biopsy is a method of obtaining a sample which is suitable for histological analysis as is required for assessment of lymphoma, prostate, diffuse liver disease (cirrhosis) or where FNAB has failed to establish a diagnosis. The biopsy needle is inserted using ultrasound guidance to the edge of the lesion before taking the sample. Automated guns are most often used to take the sample. The throw of the biopsy needle varies – this is the distance (once fired) the needle advances into the lesion.

7

Pre-procedure checks should include platelets, INR and any history of bleeding disorders. Platelets of below 50 and an INR of above 1.3/1.4 are contraindication to most core biopsies. Hypertension has been shown to increase the risk of haemorrhage following renal biopsy. Ascites is a contraindication to liver biopsy. Local sepsis may be a relative contraindication.

Complications of biopsy

- Haemorrhage.

- Infection – local or distant sites (prosthetic heart valve, joint replacement at increased risk with contaminated sites such as prostate biopsy).

- Damage to local structures, e.g. pneumothorax.

- A–V fistula (renal biopsy).

Question 3

44-year-old patient with extensive burns complicated by sepsis (Figs 7.18 and 7.19).
Ventilated on intensive care unit.
Fever, leukocytosis elevated liver enzymes and bilirubin.

- What is the diagnosis?

- What are the main complications?

- What are the treatment options?

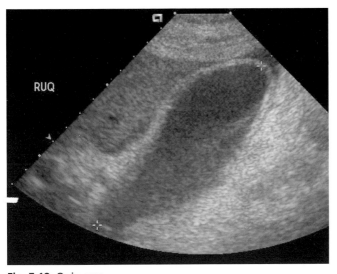

Fig. 7.18 Quiz case.

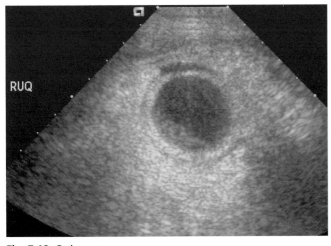

Fig. 7.19 Quiz case.

Answer

Acalculous cholecystitis

Acalculous cholecystitis is gall bladder inflammation in the absence of gall bladder calculi. It is most frequently seen in patients who are hospitalised and are acutely unwell. Risk factors include:

- severe medical illness,

- post-surgical patients,

- burns,

- trauma,

- parenteral nutrition,

- ventilation,

- prolonged fasting.

As can be seen from the list above, the risk factors are often fulfilled by patients on intensive care units. Clinical presentation may be non-specific with fever, pain (either right upper quadrant or generalised abdominal pain), leukocytosis and elevated liver enzymes or bilirubin. A small proportion of patients with acalculous cholecystitis are made up of outpatients and children. Diagnosis is more straightforward in this group. On the intensive care unit, it is a difficult diagnosis to make both clinically and radiologically. Delay in diagnosis and the related/predisposing conditions mean that it is associated with a high degree of morbidity and complications. Complications include gall bladder perforation, gangrene and emphysematous cholecystitis.

Ultrasound features include gall bladder wall thickening, gall bladder wall oedema, pericholecystic fluid, intramural gas, gall bladder distention and an ultrasonographic murphys sign. Several of the ultrasound features are non-specific – such as gall bladder wall thickening which can be seen with other conditions, e.g. hypoalbuminemic states and heart failure. Early follow-up looking for interval change can be helpful if the diagnosis is in doubt. CT is an alternative imaging modality, but is clearly less portable.

Treatment options

- Open cholecystectomy.

- Laparoscopic cholecystectomy.

- Percutaneous cholecystostomy (see Fig. 7.20).

- Percutaneous aspiration.

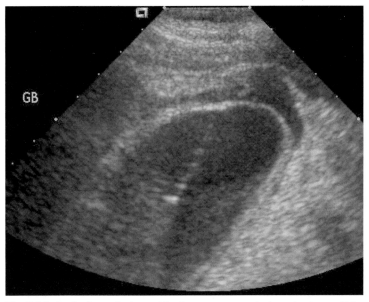

Fig. 7.20 Acalculous cholecystitis. Percutaneous cholecystostomy. Using local anaesthesia at the bedside, with ultrasound guidance a drainage catheter can be placed into the gall bladder. A locking pigtail drain can be placed as either a one-step trocar insertion or with serial dilation over a wire. A transhepatic route may reduce the risk of inadvertant drain movement. Note the echoes from the needle.

Index